Endometriosis Cookbook

Delicious recipes to nourish the body and reduce inflammation

SAVANNAH GRACE

Copyright © 2023 by Savannah Grace.

This book is a work of nonfiction. The names, characters, places, and incidents are products of the author's imagination or are used fictitiously. Any resemblance to actual events, locales, or persons, living or dead, is entirely coincidental.

Table of Contents

Introduction

Understanding Endometriosis

What is Endometriosis?

Many women who are of reproductive age suffer from the illness known as endometriosis. When endometrial-like tissue forms outside the uterus, on the ovaries, fallopian tubes, bladder, colon, or other pelvic organs, it is called endometrial dysplasia. This tissue bleeds during menstrual cycles and reacts to hormonal changes, but it cannot leave the body like regular endometrium does. Inflammation, discomfort, scarring, and occasionally infertility may result from this.

Pelvic pain is the primary sign of endometriosis, particularly during menstruation, sexual activity, or bowel movements. Heavy or irregular bleeding, exhaustion, bloating, nausea, and trouble conceiving are possible additional symptoms. Some endometriosis sufferers, however, simply experience minor symptoms or none at all. The degree of the ailment is not necessarily indicated by the intensity of the symptoms.

While some women experience little pain from a large amount of endometriosis tissue, others have tremendous agony from a tiny amount of tissue.

Although the precise etiology of endometriosis is unknown, a number of variables, including genetics, immune system abnormalities, retrograde menstruation (the movement of menstrual blood back into the fallopian tubes), or environmental pollutants, may be involved. Although endometriosis cannot be cured, there are therapies that can help control the symptoms and enhance quality of life. Hormonal therapy, surgery, supplemental therapies, and opioids are available as treatment options. The patient's objectives, such as pain relief, maintaining fertility, or preventing recurrence, will determine the course of treatment.

A prevalent and long-lasting ailment that can impact women's physical, emotional, and social health is endometriosis. If you experience endometriosis symptoms, it's critical to consult a doctor because prompt diagnosis and treatment can enhance results and minimize side effects. Additionally, a number of groups and organizations that promote endometriosis awareness and research can provide you with information and support.

Symptoms and Diagnosis

Roughly 10% of women who are of reproductive age suffer from the common condition endometriosis. This happens when endometrial tissue, which lines the interior of the uterus usually, develops outside of it in other areas of the abdomen or pelvis. This tissue bleeds during menstrual cycles and reacts to hormonal changes, but it cannot leave the body like regular endometrium does. Inflammation, scarring, adhesions, and cysts may result from this, causing persistent pain and infertility in the afflicted areas.

Pelvic pain, particularly during periods, ovulation, sex, bowel movements, or urine, is the primary symptom of endometriosis. Pain may be mild, moderate, or severe, and it may be continuous or sporadic. In addition, some women report having exhaustion, nausea, bloating, heavy or irregular bleeding, or digestive issues. Some endometriosis sufferers, however, don't exhibit any symptoms at all or don't know they have the illness until they experience difficulty conceiving.

Endometriosis cannot be definitively diagnosed because there is no test for it. The symptoms can be mistaken for those of other illnesses, including interstitial cystitis, pelvic inflammatory disease, ovarian cysts, and irritable bowel syndrome. Only a laparoscopy, a minimally invasive procedure that enables the physician to look into the pelvis and take tissue samples for biopsy, can definitively determine the existence and degree of endometriosis. Additional tests, including an MRI, ultrasound, or pelvic exam, can help rule out other possible reasons of pain or raise the chance of endometriosis, but they cannot definitively identify it.

The course of treatment for endometriosis is determined by the patient's preferences and goals, the severity of the disease, and the degree of symptoms. Hormonal therapy, surgery, or a mix of these are the available alternatives. The treatment's objectives are to lessen discomfort, lessen inflammation, stop the formation of new endometriosis tissue, and maintain or increase fertility. Although endometriosis cannot be cured, many women can enhance their quality of life and fulfill their reproductive objectives with appropriate therapy.

Treatment Options and Lifestyle Management

The degree of the disease, the patient's age, the desire to become pregnant, and the intensity of the symptoms all affect how endometriosis is treated. Relieving pain, lowering inflammation, stopping the disease's progression, and maintaining or restoring fertility are the main objectives of treatment. Among the available treatments are:

Pharmacological treatment: This entails taking drugs that inhibit the hormone estrogen, which promotes the formation of endometriosis tissue, either by inhibiting its synthesis or action. Oral contraceptives, progestins, aromatase inhibitors, gonadotropin-releasing hormone (GnRH) agonists, and selective progesterone receptor modulators (SPRMs) are some of these drugs. These drugs have adverse effects that include mood swings, weight gain, hot flashes, decreased libido, and bone loss. However, they can also lessen pain and bleeding. They are not appropriate for ladies who wish to get pregnant because they are also a form of contraception.

Surgical treatment: A laparoscopy or laparotomy is used to remove or destroy endometriosis tissue. Laparoscopy is a minimally invasive procedure that involves making tiny incisions in order to reach the pelvis using a thin tube equipped with a camera and equipment. A bigger abdominal incision is necessary for a laparotomy, a more invasive surgical procedure. Conservative surgery involves preserving the uterus and ovaries, while radical surgery involves removing the uterus, ovaries, and fallopian tubes. Surgery carries some dangers, including bleeding, adhesion development, infection, and organ damage, but it can also reduce pain and increase fertility. Endometriosis cannot be cured by surgery, and the condition may return after the procedure.

Assisted reproductive technology (ART): This refers to the use of methods to help endometriosis-affected women become pregnant, such as intrauterine insemination (IUI) or in vitro fertilization (IVF). Bypassing the effects of endometriosis on the uterus, fallopian tubes, and ovaries, ART can improve the likelihood of becoming pregnant. ART is costly, time-consuming, and emotionally taxing, though. Additionally, it may result in ectopic pregnancy, ovarian hyperstimulation syndrome, and multiple pregnancies.

Endometriosis Management via Lifestyle

Women with endometriosis can benefit from lifestyle management in addition to medical or surgical treatment in order to better manage their illness and enhance their overall health. Among the methods for managing one's lifestyle are:

Exercise: For women with endometriosis, regular physical activity can lessen pain, inflammation, stress, and sadness. In addition, blood circulation, muscle strength, and bone health can all be enhanced by exercise. It is advised to engage in moderate aerobic exercise for at least 30 minutes, three times a week, such as swimming, cycling, or walking.

Diet: Endometriosis sufferers' immune systems, hormone balances, and general health can all be supported by a well-balanced and nourishing diet. Increased consumption of fruits, vegetables, whole grains, lean proteins, and omega-3 fatty acids are advised, whereas decreased consumption of refined carbohydrates, trans fats, saturated fats, caffeine, and alcohol is advised.

Certain foods, such green tea, flaxseed, and soy, may have anti-estrogenic or anti-inflammatory properties that help endometriosis sufferers.

Stress management: By impairing the immune system, hormonal balance, and pain perception, long-term stress can exacerbate endometriosis symptoms and accelerate its progression. Women with endometriosis can benefit from stress management strategies such as breathing exercises, yoga, meditation, relaxation, and cognitive-behavioral therapy to help them manage their illness and lower their stress levels.

Support: For many women, having endometriosis can be difficult and isolated. Women with endometriosis can get emotional, practical, and informational assistance by sharing their experiences, feelings, and worries with family, friends, partners, health professionals, or support groups. Support can also provide endometriosis-affected women a sense of empowerment, hope, and motivation to take control of their illness and achieve their objectives.

Chapter 1:

The Role of Nutrition in Managing Endometriosis

Importance of Diet in Alleviating Symptoms

It is unclear what exactly causes endometriosis, although a number of things, including hormone imbalance, immunological system dysfunction, environmental pollutants, and heredity, may play a role in its onset and spread. Among these, nutrition can significantly affect intestinal health, inflammation, and estrogen levels, all of which can worsen endometriosis symptoms.

An important aspect of endometriosis is inflammation, which supports the disease's growth and survival as well as the pain and discomfort that patients experience. Depending on the kinds and amounts of foods ingested, diet can either promote or decrease inflammation. Foods like red meat, processed meat, dairy, added sugars, refined carbs, and alcohol can all cause inflammation. These meals have the potential to increase the synthesis of prostaglandins, oxidative stress, and pro-inflammatory cytokines, all of which can exacerbate endometriosis symptoms. Conversely, diets high in antioxidants, whole grains, legumes, nuts, seeds, and fatty fish can help lower inflammation. These foods can supply fiber, polyphenols, antioxidants, and omega-3 fatty acids, which can regulate the immune system and reduce inflammation.

Since estrogen promotes the development and multiplication of tissue that resembles the endometrium, it is another element that may have an impact on endometriosis. Estrogen synthesis, metabolism, and excretion can all be impacted by diet. Animal products, particularly those containing hormones or pesticides, soy products, and alcohol are foods that can raise estrogen levels. These foods have the potential to resemble or contain estrogen, or to obstruct its excretion and breakdown. Fruits, vegetables, whole grains, legumes, and cruciferous vegetables like kale, broccoli, cauliflower, and cabbage are examples of diets high in fiber that help suppress estrogen levels. Either by binding and eliminating excess estrogen from the body or by supplying phytoestrogens, which are less potent than estrogen, these foods can help control the body's activity.

Another factor that nutrition can affect is gut health, which can have an impact on endometriosis. Inflammation, hormone levels, and immune system performance can all be impacted by the gut microbiome, which is the assembly of bacteria and other microorganisms that reside in the digestive tract. Because different foods can either promote or prevent the growth of specific bacteria, diet can have an impact on the variety and composition of the gut microbiome. Beneficial bacteria that can metabolize estrogen, create anti-inflammatory compounds, and influence the immune system are prevalent and diverse in a healthy gut microbiome. Eating prebiotic foods like garlic, onion, asparagus, and bananas, as well as probiotic foods like yogurt, kefir, sauerkraut, and kimchi, can help maintain a healthy gut microbiome by supplying beneficial bacteria and their food sources.

Finally, by regulating inflammation, estrogen levels, and intestinal health, food can be a significant factor in reducing the symptoms associated with endometriosis. A diet low in animal products, particularly red meat, processed meat, dairy products, and alcohol, and high in plant-based foods, such as fruits, vegetables, whole grains, legumes, nuts, seeds, and fatty fish, can help lessen the pain, inflammation, and infertility brought on by endometriosis. An individualized diet that caters to the specific requirements and inclinations of every endometriosis sufferer can also enhance their overall health and well-being.

Foods to Avoid and Foods to Include

Foods to avoid

Certain foods may make symptoms of endometriosis worse by elevating estrogen levels, causing intestinal dysbiosis, or inflaming the body. These dishes consist of:

Trans fats: Found in fried, processed, and fast food, trans fats can elevate prostaglandins, oxidative stress, and inflammation, all of which exacerbate endometriosis pain and bleeding.

Red meat: Either by the provision of exogenous hormones or pesticides, or through disruption of its excretion and metabolism, red meat can raise estrogen levels. By raising arachidonic acid, a precursor of pro-inflammatory prostaglandins, red meat can also exacerbate oxidative stress and inflammation.

Gluten: In certain individuals, particularly those with celiac disease or gluten sensitivity, gluten, a protein present in wheat, barley, and rye, can cause an immunological reaction and inflammation. According to one study, removing gluten from their diet reduced pain for 75% of endometriosis-affected women.

Foods high in fermentable carbohydrates, or FODMAPs, can make you feel bloated, gassy, and uncomfortable in your digestive tract. This is especially true if you have small intestinal bacterial overgrowth (SIBO) or irritable bowel syndrome (IBS). A low-FODMAP diet, which can enhance gut health and lower inflammation, may be beneficial for some women with endometriosis who also have SIBO or IBS.

Alcohol: Alcohol can raise estrogen levels by preventing the liver from breaking it down and eliminating it. In addition to depleting nutrients necessary for hormonal balance and detoxification, alcohol can also increase prostaglandins, inflammation, and oxidative stress.

Foods to include

Certain foods can help alleviate the symptoms of endometriosis by lowering inflammation, estrogen levels, or dysbiosis in the gut. These dishes consist of:

Fiber: Fiber maintains a healthy gut flora, which influences the immune system and metabolizes estrogen, and it can help bind and eliminate excess estrogen from the body. Foods high in fiber include whole grains, legumes, nuts, seeds, and fruits and vegetables.

Omega-3 fats: These fats have the ability to lower prostaglandins and inflammation while also influencing gene expression and estrogen receptor function. Fatty fish like salmon, sardines, and tuna as well as nuts and seeds like flaxseed, chia seeds, and walnuts contain omega-3 fats.

Cruciferous vegetables: Due to their phytochemical content, which can alter estrogen synthesis, metabolism, and excretion, cruciferous vegetables—such as broccoli, cauliflower, cabbage, and kale—can help control estrogen levels. They can also help women with endometriosis by supplying antioxidants, fiber, and anti-inflammatory chemicals.

Probiotics and prebiotics: Beneficial bacteria that can colonize the gut and enhance its health and function are known as probiotics. Probiotic dietary sources include fructooligosaccharides (FOS) and inulin, which are known as prebiotics. Prebiotics and probiotics have been shown to improve estrogen metabolism and excretion, lower inflammation, and balance the gut microbiota. Kimchi, sauerkraut, kefir, and yogurt are examples of probiotic-rich foods. Bananas, asparagus, garlic, and onions are examples of prebiotic foods.

Impact of Diet on Hormonal Balance

One essential hormone for proper functioning is estrogen, which you need in some amounts. However, excessive estrogen can exacerbate endometriosis symptoms by promoting the development and multiplication of tissue that resembles the endometrium. Estrogen synthesis, metabolism, and excretion can all be impacted by diet. Among the food components that can raise estrogen levels are:

Animal items, including eggs, dairy, and red meat that may include hormones or pesticides. These goods may resemble estrogen, contain it, or prevent the liver from breaking it down and getting rid of it.

Soy items, including edamame, tofu, and soy milk. Phytoestrogens, or plant chemicals with properties akin to those of estrogen, are present in these items. Soy's impact on endometriosis is debatable, though. While some research contends that soy may help by rivaling estrogen for receptor sites, other studies contend that soy may worsen the condition by raising estrogen levels.

Alcohol, which may hinder the liver's capacity to break down and eliminate estrogen. Alcohol can also accelerate the enzyme aromatase's conversion of androgens to estrogens.

Dietary components that can lower estrogen levels include:

Fiber: It has the ability to bind and expel excess estrogen from the body through stools. Foods high in fiber include whole grains, legumes, nuts, seeds, and fruits and vegetables.

Cruciferous vegetables, which include kale, broccoli, cauliflower, and cabbage. These vegetables include phytochemicals that have the ability to alter the synthesis, metabolism, and excretion of estrogens through the cytochrome P450 enzyme system. They can also help women with endometriosis by supplying antioxidants, fiber, and anti-inflammatory chemicals.

Flaxseed, a plant high in lignans, a kind of phytoestrogen that can limit the conversion of androgens to estrogens by inhibiting the enzyme aromatase. Omega-3 fatty acids, which can modify estrogen receptor function and gene expression and lower prostaglandins and inflammation, are also found in flaxseed.

Building a Balanced Endometriosis Diet

Incorporating Essential Nutrients

The following are a few vital nutrients that can help women with endometriosis:

Iron: The mineral iron is needed to make red blood cells, which are responsible for distributing oxygen throughout the body. Anemia, which can exacerbate endometriosis symptoms including weakness, exhaustion, and heavy bleeding, can be brought on by an iron shortage. Endometriosis patients need to get adequate iron from their diet, which can be obtained from foods like lean meat, chicken, fish, eggs, beans, lentils, and fortified cereals, as well as supplements if prescribed by a physician.

Vitamin B12: This vitamin is necessary for the production of red blood cells, the upkeep of nerve cells, and the creation of DNA. Anemia and neurological issues including tingling, numbness, and memory loss can also be brought on by a vitamin B12 shortage. Vitamin B12 deficiency is a possibility for endometriosis-afflicted women, particularly in those with intestinal conditions like Crohn's disease or celiac disease that affect the absorption of the vitamin. Animal items such meat, poultry, fish, eggs, and dairy products, as well as fortified foods like cereals, soy milk, and nutritional yeast, are the primary sources of vitamin B12. When dealing with endometriosis, women should make sure they are getting enough vitamin B12 from their diet and, if necessary, supplements.

Vitamin D: This vitamin is crucial for controlling the body's levels of calcium and phosphorus, both of which are necessary for strong bones. Along with its immunomodulatory and anti-inflammatory properties, vitamin D may also help lessen the pain and inflammation brought on by endometriosis. In addition to being produced by the skin when exposed to sunshine, vitamin D can also be consumed through fortified foods like milk, orange juice, and cereals, as well as meals high in fat, including cheese, egg yolks, and fatty fish. But a lot of people, particularly in the winter or in places with little solar exposure, lack vitamin D.

Endometriosis patients should have their vitamin D levels tested by a physician and, if needed, take supplements.

Omega-3 fatty acids: These polyunsaturated fats provide antioxidant and anti-inflammatory qualities that may help lessen the discomfort and inflammation brought on by endometriosis. Aside from their ability to influence gene expression and estrogen receptor activation, omega-3 fatty acids may also have an impact on the development and survival of endometrial-like tissue. Nuts and seeds like walnuts, chia seeds, and flaxseed, as well as fatty seafood like tuna, salmon, and sardines, contain omega-3 fatty acids. If recommended by their doctor, women with endometriosis should take fish oil supplements or try to eat two or more servings of fatty fish each week.

Magnesium: The body uses magnesium for over 300 enzymatic processes, such as nerve and muscle transmission, energy synthesis, and muscular contraction. A lack of magnesium can exacerbate endometriosis symptoms by causing discomfort, cramps, and spasms in the muscles. Additionally, magnesium has the ability to calm the uterine smooth muscles, which may lessen monthly cramps and bleeding. Whole grains, legumes, nuts, seeds, and dark chocolate are good sources of magnesium.

If necessary, endometriosis-affected women should take magnesium supplements or get enough of it through food.

Creating Meal Plans for Symptom Relief

Creating meal plans for symptom relief of endometriosis can help women follow a balanced and varied diet that is rich in plant-based foods, especially fruits, vegetables, whole grains, legumes, nuts, and seeds, and low in animal products, especially red meat, dairy products, and alcohol. A meal plan can also help women incorporate foods that can benefit endometriosis, such as omega-3 fatty acids, fiber, cruciferous vegetables, probiotics, and prebiotics, and avoid foods that can worsen endometriosis, such as trans fats, gluten, high-FODMAP foods, and caffeine.

A sample 7-day meal plan for symptom relief of endometriosis is as follows:

Day 1

Breakfast: Oatmeal with almond milk, flaxseed, blueberries, and walnuts
Snack: Apple with almond butter
Lunch: Kale and quinoa salad with chickpeas, cherry tomatoes, avocado, and lemon dressing
Snack: Carrot sticks with hummus
Dinner: Baked salmon with roasted broccoli and brown rice

Day 2

Breakfast: Scrambled eggs with spinach and whole wheat toast
Snack: Banana with sunflower seed butter
Lunch: Lentil and vegetable soup with whole wheat pita bread
Snack: Greek yogurt with strawberries and granola
Dinner: Spaghetti squash with turkey meatballs and marinara sauce

Day 3

Breakfast: Smoothie with almond milk, spinach, banana, and chia seeds
Snack: Trail mix with almonds, raisins, and dark chocolate
Lunch: Chicken and vegetable stir-fry with brown rice noodles

Snack: Celery sticks with peanut butter

Dinner: Roasted cauliflower and chickpea curry with basmati rice

Day 4

Breakfast: Whole wheat pancakes with maple syrup and fresh berries

Snack: Orange with cashews

Lunch: Turkey and avocado sandwich on whole wheat bread with lettuce and tomato

Snack: Edamame with sea salt

Dinner: Vegetable and bean chili with cornbread

Day 5

Breakfast: Muesli with soy milk, dried fruits, and nuts

Snack: Kiwi with pistachios

Lunch: Spinach and mushroom quiche with green salad

Snack: Cottage cheese with pineapple and sunflower seeds

Dinner: Tofu and vegetable skewers with couscous and tzatziki sauce

Day 6

Breakfast: French toast with almond butter and banana
Snack: Pear with cheese
Lunch: Black bean and sweet potato burrito with salsa and guacamole
Snack: Popcorn with nutritional yeast
Dinner: Roasted chicken with roasted potatoes and asparagus

Day 7

Breakfast: Chia pudding with coconut milk, mango, and coconut flakes
Snack: Grapefruit with walnuts
Lunch: Vegetable and cheese frittata with whole wheat muffin
Snack: Kefir with raspberries and honey
Dinner: Vegetable and tofu lasagna with green salad

Tips for Grocery Shopping and Meal Preparation

Nutrition is a key factor in the management of endometriosis since it can supply vital nutrients that support immunological response, hormonal balance, and general health.

Additionally, it can aid in lowering intestinal dysbiosis, inflammation, and estrogen levels—all of which are linked to endometriosis symptoms. Endometriosis-related discomfort, inflammation, and infertility may be lessened with a diet high in plant-based foods, including fruits, vegetables, whole grains, legumes, nuts, and seeds, and low in animal products, particularly dairy, alcohol, and red meat.

But maintaining a balanced diet can be difficult, particularly when it comes to meal planning and grocery shopping. The following advice can help to make it simpler and more pleasurable:

Make a plan: You may save time, money, and energy by organizing your meals for the coming week. Your diet plans may be derailed by impulsive purchases and eating out, which it can also help you avoid.

Shop wisely: Purchasing the healthiest, freshest, and most reasonably priced goods for your diet is a sign of smart shopping. Here are some pointers for frugal shopping: - Look throughout the supermarket for fresh produce, dairy items, lean meats, seafood, and eggs. Steer clear of the center aisles where processed, packaged, and junk food are found.

Whenever feasible, purchase organic, hormone- and pesticide-free foods; this is especially important for animal products and thin-skinned fruits and vegetables like spinach, apples, and strawberries. These foods may imitate or contain estrogen, which might exacerbate the symptoms of endometriosis.

Purchase goods in quantity, particularly necessities like grains, beans, nuts, seeds, and spices. These meals can save you money and grocery shop excursions because they are long-lasting.

Purchase fruits and vegetables in frozen, canned, or dry form, especially if they are too costly or out of season. These foods can still be convenient and adaptable for cooking, and they can still include fiber and nutrients.

Cook wisely: This refers to arranging your food to optimize flavor, nutrition, and ease of use. Cooking in batches and freezing or refrigerating leftovers are some sensible cooking strategies. This can guarantee that you always have a nutritious meal ready to eat while also saving you time and effort.

When cooking, use healthy fats like avocado, coconut, or olive oil; steer clear of trans fats like vegetables, margarine, or shortening. Trans fats can have the opposite effect of healthy fats in terms of lowering inflammation and regulating estrogen levels.

Instead of using salt, sugar, or artificial additives in your cooking, try using herbs, spices, and condiments like coconut aminos, ginger, garlic, turmeric, cinnamon, lemon, and vinegar. While salt, sugar, and artificial additives can raise estrogen levels, induce inflammation, and cause gut dysbiosis, herbs, spices, and condiments can enhance flavor, antioxidants, and anti-inflammatory chemicals in your food.

Use other cooking techniques instead of frying, microwaving, or boiling food, such as steaming, baking, roasting, or grilling. The taste, texture, and nutrient content of your food can all be influenced by different cooking techniques, some of which may be healthier than others. For instance, steaming helps retain the vitamins and minerals in vegetables, but frying can produce unhealthy substances like acrylamide.

Chapter 2:

Breakfast Delights

Recipe 1:

Anti-Inflammatory Blueberry Hemp Seed Smoothie

Ingredients:

- 1 1/4 cup (140 g) frozen blueberries (or other frozen berry of choice)
- 2 tbsp (22 g) hemp seeds
- 1 serving (30 g) vanilla plant-based protein powder
- 1/2 cup packed (30 g), fresh spinach or kale
- 1 tsp spirulina or chlorella powder
- 1 1/4 unsweetened plant-based milk of choice
- 1/4 tsp holy basil powder (optional)

Preparation:

- Add all the ingredients to a blender and blend until smooth and creamy.
- Enjoy a refreshing and nourishing breakfast.

Nutritional value (per serving):

- Calories: 375 kcal
- Protein: 25 g
- Fat: 15 g
- Carbohydrates: 40 g
- Fiber: 10 g
- Sugar: 23 g

Cooking time: 5 minutes

Recipe 2:

Superfoods Detox Smoothie

Ingredients:
- 2 cups freshly squeezed orange juice, or equal quantity peeled and pitted oranges
- 1 unpeeled, pitted apple
- 1 ripe banana
- 3 tablespoons goji berries
- 1 teaspoon turmeric
- A pinch of pepper
- 1 teaspoon cinnamon
- 2 tablespoons tahini (you can up this to 4 tablespoons or even replace with almond butter)
- 3 brazil nuts

- 2 teaspoons fresh grated ginger
- 3 teaspoons chia seeds

Preparation:
- Soak the goji berries in water for 10 minutes, then drain and rinse.
- Add all the ingredients to a blender and blend until smooth and frothy.
- Enjoy a detoxifying and energizing breakfast.

Nutritional value (per serving):
- Calories: 495 kcal
- Protein: 12 g
- Fat: 23 g
- Carbohydrates: 68 g
- Fiber: 14 g
- Sugar: 43 g

Cooking time: 15 minutes

Recipe 3:

Easy Anti-Inflammatory Green Smoothie

Ingredients:

- 2 cups spinach
- 2 cups water
- 1 cup mango
- 1 cup pineapple
- 2 bananas, Use at least one frozen fruit to chill your smoothie. We often use frozen mangos and bananas for our green smoothies.

Preparation:
- Add the spinach and water to a blender and blend until smooth.
- Add the rest of the ingredients and blend again until creamy and smooth.
- Enjoy a simple and delicious breakfast.

Nutritional value (per serving):
- Calories: 240 kcal
- Protein: 3 g
- Fat: 1 g
- Carbohydrates: 60 g
- Fiber: 7 g
- Sugar: 42 g

Cooking time: 5 minutes

Recipe 4:

Anti-Inflammatory Healing Bowl with Sweet Potatoes, Turmeric and Kale

Ingredients:
- 2 sweet potatoes, cubed (roughly 3 cups cubed)
- 2 T coconut oil, divided
- 1 red bell pepper, diced
- 1 red onion, diced
- 3 garlic cloves, minced
- 1 t ground turmeric
- ½ t pepper
- 2 cups chopped kale, ribs removed
- Salt to taste
- 2 servings of plant-based protein of choice, such as tofu, tempeh, or beans
- 1 avocado, sliced lengthwise

Preparation:
- Preheat the oven to 375°F (190°C) and line a baking sheet with parchment paper.
- Toss the sweet potatoes with 1 T of coconut oil and spread them on the prepared baking sheet. Bake for 25 minutes, flipping halfway through, until tender and golden.

- In a large skillet over medium-high heat, heat the remaining 1 T of coconut oil and sauté the bell pepper, onion, garlic, turmeric, and pepper for 15 minutes, stirring occasionally, until soft and caramelized.
- Add the kale and a pinch of salt and cook for another 5 minutes, until wilted and bright green.
- In a separate skillet over medium-high heat, cook your plant-based protein of choice according to the package directions, seasoning with salt and pepper as desired.
- To serve, divide the sweet potatoes, kale mixture, and protein among two bowls. Top with avocado slices and enjoy a warm and comforting breakfast.

Nutritional value (per serving):
- Calories: 570 kcal
- Protein: 20 g
- Fat: 32 g
- Carbohydrates: 60 g
- Fiber: 18 g
- Sugar: 18 g

Cooking time: 45 minutes

Recipe 5:

Paleo Avocado Sweet Potato Toast Recipe

Ingredients:
- 2 large sweet potatoes, ends removed and sliced lengthwise into ¼-inch (0.65 cm) thick slices
- Salt, to taste
- 2 large avocados, mashed
- 1/4 cup (60 ml) Paleo pizza sauce or tomato sauce
- Optional toppings: cherry tomatoes, basil leaves, hemp seeds, nutritional yeast, etc.

Preparation:
- Preheat the oven to 400°F (200°C) and line a baking sheet with parchment paper.
- Arrange the sweet potato slices on the prepared baking sheet and sprinkle with salt. Bake for 15 minutes, flip, and bake for another 10 minutes, until tender and slightly crisp.
- To serve, spread the mashed avocado on each sweet potato slice, then top with pizza sauce or tomato sauce and your optional toppings of choice. Enjoy a savory and satisfying breakfast.

Nutritional value (per serving):
- Calories: 320 kcal
- Protein: 6 g
- Fat: 20 g
- Carbohydrates: 36 g
- Fiber: 14 g
- Sugar: 12 g

Cooking time: 30 minutes

Recipe 6:

Cinnamon and Raisin Bread Pudding

Ingredients:
- 4 slices of gluten-free bread, cubed
- 2 cups of unsweetened almond milk
- 2 tablespoons of maple syrup
- 2 teaspoons of vanilla extract
- 1 teaspoon of cinnamon
- 1/4 teaspoon of nutmeg
- 1/4 cup of raisins
- 2 tablespoons of chopped walnuts

Preparation:
- Preheat the oven to 180°C (350°F) and grease a baking dish.
- In a large bowl, whisk together the almond milk, maple syrup, vanilla, cinnamon, and nutmeg.
- Add the bread cubes and raisins and toss to coat well.
- Transfer the mixture to the prepared baking dish and sprinkle with walnuts.
- Bake for 25 to 30 minutes, until golden and set.
- Enjoy a warm and cozy breakfast.

Nutritional value (per serving):
- Calories: 260 kcal
- Protein: 6 g
- Fat: 9 g
- Carbohydrates: 41 g
- Fiber: 4 g
- Sugar: 19 g

Cooking time: 40 minutes

Recipe 7:

Quinoa Breakfast Bowl with Berries and Nuts

Ingredients:
- 1 cup of quinoa, rinsed and drained
- 2 cups of water
- A pinch of salt
- 1/4 cup of unsweetened almond milk
- 2 tablespoons of maple syrup
- 1/4 teaspoon of vanilla extract
- 1/4 teaspoon of cinnamon
- 1 cup of fresh or frozen mixed berries
- 1/4 cup of chopped almonds

Preparation:
- In a small saucepan, bring the quinoa, water, and salt to a boil. Reduce the heat and simmer, covered, for 15 to 20 minutes, until the quinoa is fluffy and the water is absorbed.
- Fluff the quinoa with a fork and stir in the almond milk, maple syrup, vanilla, and cinnamon.
- Divide the quinoa among two bowls and top with berries and almonds.
- Enjoy a nutritious and filling breakfast.

Nutritional value (per serving):
- Calories: 410 kcal
- Protein: 12 g
- Fat: 12 g
- Carbohydrates: 66 g
- Fiber: 9 g
- Sugar: 23 g

Cooking time: 25 minutes

Recipe 8:

Banana and Date Cake

Ingredients:
- 2 ripe bananas, mashed
- 1/4 cup of coconut oil, melted
- 1/4 cup of maple syrup
- 1 teaspoon of vanilla extract
- 2 cups of almond flour
- 1 teaspoon of baking soda
- 1/4 teaspoon of salt
- 1/4 cup of chopped dates

Preparation:
- Preheat the oven to 180°C (350°F) and line a loaf pan with parchment paper.
- In a large bowl, whisk together the bananas, coconut oil, maple syrup, and vanilla.
- In a separate bowl, whisk together the almond flour, baking soda, and salt.
- Add the dry ingredients to the wet ingredients and stir to combine. Fold in the dates.
- Pour the batter into the prepared loaf pan and smooth the top.

- Bake for 35 to 40 minutes, until a toothpick inserted comes out clean.
- Let the cake cool slightly before slicing and serving.
- Enjoy a moist and delicious breakfast.

Nutritional value (per serving):
- Calories: 280 kcal
- Protein: 6 g
- Fat: 18 g
- Carbohydrates: 26 g
- Fiber: 4 g
- Sugar: 17 g

Cooking time: 50 minutes

Recipe 9:

Buckwheat Berry Pie

Ingredients:
- 1 cup of buckwheat flour
- 1/4 cup of coconut oil, melted
- 2 tablespoons of maple syrup
- A pinch of salt
- 2 cups of mixed berries, fresh or frozen
- 2 tablespoons of cornstarch

- 2 tablespoons of water
- 2 tablespoons of lemon juice
- 2 tablespoons of coconut sugar

Preparation:
- Preheat the oven to 180°C (350°F) and grease a pie dish.
- In a medium bowl, mix together the buckwheat flour, coconut oil, maple syrup, and salt. Press the dough evenly into the bottom and sides of the prepared pie dish. Prick the dough with a fork and bake for 15 minutes, until golden and firm.
- In a small saucepan, combine the berries, cornstarch, water, lemon juice, and coconut sugar. Bring to a boil, then reduce the heat and simmer, stirring occasionally, for 10 minutes, until the berries are soft and the sauce is thickened.
- Pour the berry mixture over the crust and spread evenly.
- Bake for another 10 minutes, until bubbly.
- Let the pie cool slightly before slicing and serving.
- Enjoy a fruity and gluten-free breakfast.

Nutritional value (per serving):
- Calories: 250 kcal
- Protein: 3 g
- Fat: 12 g
- Carbohydrates: 36 g
- Fiber: 5 g

- Sugar: 18 g

Cooking time: 40 minutes

Recipe 10:

Chia Pudding with Coconut Milk, Mango, and Coconut Flakes

Ingredients:
- 1/4 cup of chia seeds
- 1 cup of coconut milk
- 2 tablespoons of maple syrup
- 1/4 teaspoon of vanilla extract
- 1/4 teaspoon of cardamom
- 1 cup of diced mango, fresh or frozen
- 2 tablespoons of coconut flakes, toasted

Preparation:
- In a small bowl, whisk together the chia seeds, coconut milk, maple syrup, vanilla, and cardamom. Refrigerate for at least 4 hours, or overnight, until thick and gel-like.
- In a small skillet over medium heat, toast the coconut flakes, stirring frequently, until golden and

crisp, about 5 minutes. Transfer to a plate and let cool.

- To serve, divide the chia pudding among two bowls and top with mango and coconut flakes.

- Enjoy a tropical and creamy breakfast.

Nutritional value (per serving):

- Calories: 400 kcal

- Protein: 7 g

- Fat: 27 g

- Carbohydrates: 39 g

- Fiber: 13 g

- Sugar: 25 g

Cooking time: 10 minutes (plus refrigeration time)

Chapter 3:

Nourishing Lunches

Recipe 1:

Mediterranean Quinoa Salad

Ingredients:
- 1 cup of quinoa, rinsed and drained
- 2 cups of vegetable broth or water
- A pinch of salt
- 2 tablespoons of lemon juice
- 2 tablespoons of olive oil
- 1/4 teaspoon of oregano
- 1/4 teaspoon of garlic powder
- 2 cups of baby spinach, chopped
- 1/4 cup of kalamata olives, pitted and sliced
- 1/4 cup of sun-dried tomatoes, chopped
- 2 tablespoons of pine nuts, toasted

Preparation:
- In a small saucepan, bring the quinoa, broth or water, and salt to a boil. Reduce the heat and

simmer, covered, for 15 to 20 minutes, until the quinoa is fluffy and the liquid is absorbed.
- In a small bowl, whisk together the lemon juice, olive oil, oregano, and garlic powder.
- In a large bowl, toss the quinoa with the spinach, olives, sun-dried tomatoes, and pine nuts. Drizzle with the dressing and toss to combine.
- Enjoy a fresh and flavorful salad.

Nutritional value (per serving):
- Calories: 360 kcal
- Protein: 10 g
- Fat: 19 g
- Carbohydrates: 42 g
- Fiber: 7 g
- Sugar: 8 g

Cooking time: 25 minutes

Recipe 2:

Roasted Vegetable and Hummus Wrap

Ingredients:

- 1 medium zucchini, sliced
- 1 medium yellow squash, sliced
- 1 medium red onion, cut into wedges
- 1 medium red bell pepper, cut into strips
- 2 tablespoons of olive oil
- Salt and pepper, to taste
- 4 gluten-free tortillas
- 1/2 cup of hummus
- 2 cups of baby spinach
- 1/4 cup of fresh parsley, chopped

Preparation:
- Preheat the oven to 200°C (400°F) and line a baking sheet with parchment paper.
- In a large bowl, toss the zucchini, squash, onion, and bell pepper with the olive oil, salt, and pepper. Spread them on the prepared baking sheet in a single layer. Roast for 25 to 30 minutes, until tender and browned, flipping halfway through.
- To assemble the wraps, spread 2 tablespoons of hummus on each tortilla. Top with spinach, roasted vegetables, and parsley. Fold the bottom edge over the filling, then fold in the sides and roll up tightly.
- Enjoy as a hearty and satisfying wrap.

Nutritional value (per serving):
- Calories: 320 kcal
- Protein: 9 g
- Fat: 16 g

- Carbohydrates: 40 g
- Fiber: 9 g
- Sugar: 11 g

Cooking time: 40 minutes

Recipe 3:

Creamy Broccoli and Cauliflower Soup

Ingredients:
- 1 tablespoon of coconut oil
- 1 medium onion, chopped
- 3 cloves of garlic, minced
- 4 cups of vegetable broth
- 4 cups of broccoli florets
- 4 cups of cauliflower florets
- 1/4 teaspoon of nutmeg
- Salt and pepper, to taste
- 1/4 cup of nutritional yeast
- 2 tablespoons of lemon juice

Preparation:
- In a large pot over medium-high heat, heat the coconut oil and sauté the onion and garlic for 10 minutes, until soft and translucent.
- Add the broth, broccoli, cauliflower, nutmeg, salt, and pepper and bring to a boil. Reduce the heat and simmer, covered, for 15 to 20 minutes, until the vegetables are tender.
- Using an immersion blender or a regular blender, puree the soup until smooth and creamy. Stir in the nutritional yeast and lemon juice.
- Enjoy as a warm and comforting soup.

Nutritional value (per serving):
- Calories: 140 kcal
- Protein: 9 g
- Fat: 5 g
- Carbohydrates: 18 g
- Fiber: 7 g
- Sugar: 7 g

Cooking time: 35 minutes

Recipe 4:

Chickpea and Avocado Salad Sandwich

Ingredients:
- 1 15-ounce can of chickpeas, drained and rinsed
- 1/4 cup of vegan mayonnaise
- 2 tablespoons of Dijon mustard
- 1/4 teaspoon of paprika
- Salt and pepper, to taste
- 8 slices of gluten-free bread, toasted
- 1 large avocado, sliced
- 4 lettuce leaves
- 1/4 cup of alfalfa sprouts

Preparation:
- In a medium bowl, mash the chickpeas with a fork or a potato masher. Add the vegan mayonnaise, mustard, paprika, salt, and pepper and mix well.
- To assemble the sandwiches, spread the chickpea mixture on four slices of bread. Top with avocado, lettuce, and sprouts. Cover with the remaining slices of bread and cut in half.
- Enjoy as a protein-packed and creamy sandwich.

Nutritional value (per serving):
- Calories: 440 kcal
- Protein: 15 g
- Fat: 21 g
- Carbohydrates: 52 g
- Fiber: 14 g
- Sugar: 9 g

Cooking time: 15 minutes

Recipe 5:

Thai Coconut Curry with Tofu and Vegetables

Ingredients:
- 1 tablespoon of coconut oil
- 1 14-ounce block of extra-firm tofu, drained, pressed, and cubed
- Salt and pepper, to taste
- 1/4 cup of red curry paste
- 1 13.5-ounce can of coconut milk
- 2 tablespoons of soy sauce or tamari
- 1 tablespoon of maple syrup
- 1 tablespoon of lime juice
- 2 cups of chopped bok choy

- 1 cup of sliced carrots
- 1 cup of sliced mushrooms
- 1/4 cup of chopped cilantro
- 2 cups of cooked brown rice

Preparation:
- In a large skillet over medium-high heat, heat the coconut oil and fry the tofu for 15 to 20 minutes, turning occasionally, until golden and crisp. Season with salt and pepper and transfer to a plate.
- In the same skillet over medium-low heat, whisk together the curry paste, coconut milk, soy sauce or tamari, maple syrup, and lime juice. Bring to a simmer and cook for 10 minutes, stirring occasionally, until slightly thickened.
- Add the bok choy, carrots, and mushrooms and cook for another 10 minutes, until the vegetables are tender.
- Stir in the cilantro and the tofu and heat through.
- Serve over brown rice and enjoy as a spicy and creamy curry.

Nutritional value (per serving):
- Calories: 520 kcal
- Protein: 18 g
- Fat: 32 g
- Carbohydrates: 47 g
- Fiber: 7 g
- Sugar: 13 g

Cooking time: 45 minutes

Recipe 6:

Mediterranean Quinoa Salad

Ingredients:
- 1 cup of quinoa, rinsed and drained
- 2 cups of vegetable broth or water
- A pinch of salt
- 2 tablespoons of lemon juice
- 2 tablespoons of olive oil
- 1/4 teaspoon of oregano
- 1/4 teaspoon of garlic powder
- 2 cups of baby spinach, chopped
- 1/4 cup of kalamata olives, pitted and sliced
- 1/4 cup of sun-dried tomatoes, chopped
- 2 tablespoons of pine nuts, toasted

Preparation:
- In a small saucepan, bring the quinoa, broth or water, and salt to a boil. Reduce the heat and simmer, covered, for 15 to 20 minutes, until the quinoa is fluffy and the liquid is absorbed.
- In a small bowl, whisk together the lemon juice, olive oil, oregano, and garlic powder.

- In a large bowl, toss the quinoa with the spinach, olives, sun-dried tomatoes, and pine nuts. Drizzle with the dressing and toss to combine.
- Enjoy a fresh and flavorful salad.

Nutritional value (per serving):
- Calories: 360 kcal
- Protein: 10 g
- Fat: 19 g
- Carbohydrates: 42 g
- Fiber: 7 g
- Sugar: 8 g

Cooking time: 25 minutes

Recipe 7:

Roasted Vegetable and Hummus Wrap

Ingredients:
- 1 medium zucchini, sliced
- 1 medium yellow squash, sliced
- 1 medium red onion, cut into wedges
- 1 medium red bell pepper, cut into strips
- 2 tablespoons of olive oil

- Salt and pepper, to taste
- 4 gluten-free tortillas
- 1/2 cup of hummus
- 2 cups of baby spinach
- 1/4 cup of fresh parsley, chopped

Preparation:
- Preheat the oven to 200°C (400°F) and line a baking sheet with parchment paper.
- In a large bowl, toss the zucchini, squash, onion, and bell pepper with the olive oil, salt, and pepper. Spread them on the prepared baking sheet in a single layer. Roast for 25 to 30 minutes, until tender and browned, flipping halfway through.
- To assemble the wraps, spread 2 tablespoons of hummus on each tortilla. Top with spinach, roasted vegetables, and parsley. Fold the bottom edge over the filling, then fold in the sides and roll up tightly.
- Enjoy as a hearty and satisfying wrap.

Nutritional value (per serving):
- Calories: 320 kcal
- Protein: 9 g
- Fat: 16 g
- Carbohydrates: 40 g
- Fiber: 9 g
- Sugar: 11 g

Cooking time: 40 minutes

Recipe 8:

Creamy Broccoli and Cauliflower Soup

Ingredients:
- 1 tablespoon of coconut oil
- 1 medium onion, chopped
- 3 cloves of garlic, minced
- 4 cups of vegetable broth
- 4 cups of broccoli florets
- 4 cups of cauliflower florets
- 1/4 teaspoon of nutmeg
- Salt and pepper, to taste
- 1/4 cup of nutritional yeast
- 2 tablespoons of lemon juice

Preparation:
- In a large pot over medium-high heat, heat the coconut oil and sauté the onion and garlic for 10 minutes, until soft and translucent.
- Add the broth, broccoli, cauliflower, nutmeg, salt, and pepper and bring to a boil. Reduce the heat and simmer, covered, for 15 to 20 minutes, until the vegetables are tender.
- Using an immersion blender or a regular blender, puree the soup until smooth and creamy. Stir in the nutritional yeast and lemon juice.

- Enjoy as a warm and comforting soup.

Nutritional value (per serving):
- Calories: 140 kcal
- Protein: 9 g
- Fat: 5 g
- Carbohydrates: 18 g
- Fiber: 7 g
- Sugar: 7 g

Cooking time: 35 minutes

Recipe 9:

Chickpea and Avocado Salad Sandwich

Ingredients:
- 1 15-ounce can of chickpeas, drained and rinsed
- 1/4 cup of vegan mayonnaise
- 2 tablespoons of Dijon mustard
- 1/4 teaspoon of paprika
- Salt and pepper, to taste
- 8 slices of gluten-free bread, toasted
- 1 large avocado, sliced
- 4 lettuce leaves

- 1/4 cup of alfalfa sprouts

Preparation:
- In a medium bowl, mash the chickpeas with a fork or a potato masher. Add the vegan mayonnaise, mustard, paprika, salt, and pepper and mix well.
- To assemble the sandwiches, spread the chickpea mixture on four slices of bread. Top with avocado, lettuce, and sprouts. Cover with the remaining slices of bread and cut in half.
- Enjoy as a protein-packed and creamy sandwich.

Nutritional value (per serving):
- Calories: 440 kcal
- Protein: 15 g
- Fat: 21 g
- Carbohydrates: 52 g
- Fiber: 14 g
- Sugar: 9 g

Cooking time: 15 minutes

Recipe 10:

Thai Coconut Curry with Tofu and Vegetables

Ingredients:
- 1 tablespoon of coconut oil
- 1 14-ounce block of extra-firm tofu, drained, pressed, and cubed
- Salt and pepper, to taste
- 1/4 cup of red curry paste
- 1 13.5-ounce can of coconut milk
- 2 tablespoons of soy sauce or tamari
- 1 tablespoon of maple syrup
- 1 tablespoon of lime juice
- 2 cups of chopped bok choy
- 1 cup of sliced carrots
- 1 cup of sliced mushrooms
- 1/4 cup of chopped cilantro
- 2 cups of cooked brown rice

Preparation:
- In a large skillet over medium-high heat, heat the coconut oil and fry the tofu for 15 to 20 minutes, turning occasionally, until golden and crisp. Season with salt and pepper and transfer to a plate.
- In the same skillet over medium-low heat, whisk together the curry paste, coconut milk, soy sauce or

tamari, maple syrup, and lime juice. Bring to a simmer and cook for 10 minutes, stirring occasionally, until slightly thickened.

- Add the bok choy, carrots, and mushrooms and cook for another 10 minutes, until the vegetables are tender.

- Stir in the cilantro and the tofu and heat through.

- Serve over brown rice and enjoy it as a spicy and creamy curry.

Nutritional value (per serving):
- Calories: 520 kcal
- Protein: 18 g
- Fat: 32 g
- Carbohydrates: 47 g
- Fiber: 7 g
- Sugar: 13 g

Cooking time: 45 minutes

Chapter 4:

Satisfying Dinners

Recipe 1:

Lentil and Mushroom Shepherd's Pie

Ingredients:
- 1 tablespoon of olive oil
- 1 onion, chopped
- 3 cloves of garlic, minced
- 2 carrots, peeled and diced
- 2 celery stalks, diced
- 2 cups of mushrooms, sliced
- 2 teaspoons of dried thyme
- 2 teaspoons of dried rosemary
- Salt and pepper, to taste
- 2 tablespoons of tomato paste
- 2 tablespoons of gluten-free soy sauce or tamari
- 2 cups of vegetable broth
- 2 cups of cooked brown or green lentils
- 2 tablespoons of cornstarch
- 4 cups of mashed potatoes (made with plant-based milk and butter)

- 2 tablespoons of nutritional yeast

Preparation:
- Preheat the oven to 180°C (350°F) and grease a 9x13 inch baking dish.
- In a large skillet over medium-high heat, heat the olive oil and sauté the onion, garlic, carrots, celery, mushrooms, thyme, rosemary, salt, and pepper for 15 to 20 minutes, until the vegetables are soft and browned.
- Stir in the tomato paste and soy sauce or tamari and cook for another 5 minutes, until well combined.
- In a small bowl, whisk together the broth, lentils, and cornstarch. Add the mixture to the skillet and bring to a boil. Reduce the heat and simmer, stirring occasionally, for 10 minutes, until the sauce is thickened.
- Transfer the lentil and mushroom mixture to the prepared baking dish and spread it evenly. Spoon the mashed potatoes over the top and sprinkle with nutritional yeast.
- Bake for 25 to 30 minutes, until the potatoes are golden and the filling is bubbly.
- Enjoy a hearty and comforting dinner.

Nutritional value (per serving):
- Calories: 360 kcal
- Protein: 15 g

- Fat: 7 g
- Carbohydrates: 60 g
- Fiber: 15 g
- Sugar: 9 g

Cooking time: 60 minutes

Recipe 2:

Roasted Vegetable and Quinoa Buddha Bowl

Ingredients:
- 2 cups of cooked quinoa
- 2 cups of broccoli florets
- 2 cups of cauliflower florets
- 2 cups of Brussels sprouts, halved
- 2 tablespoons of olive oil
- Salt and pepper, to taste
- 1/4 cup of tahini
- 2 tablespoons of lemon juice
- 2 tablespoons of water
- 1 teaspoon of maple syrup
- 1/4 teaspoon of garlic powder
- 1/4 teaspoon of cumin
- 4 cups of baby spinach

- 1/4 cup of pumpkin seeds

Preparation:
- Preheat the oven to 200°C (400°F) and line two baking sheets with parchment paper.
- In a large bowl, toss the broccoli, cauliflower, and Brussels sprouts with the olive oil, salt, and pepper. Spread them on the prepared baking sheets in a single layer. Roast for 25 to 30 minutes, until tender and browned, flipping halfway through.
- In a small bowl, whisk together the tahini, lemon juice, water, maple syrup, garlic powder, and cumin. Adjust the consistency and seasoning as needed.
- To serve, divide the quinoa among four bowls and top with spinach, roasted vegetables, and pumpkin seeds. Drizzle with the tahini dressing and enjoy a nutritious and satisfying dinner.

Nutritional value (per serving):
- Calories: 420 kcal
- Protein: 16 g
- Fat: 22 g
- Carbohydrates: 46 g
- Fiber: 12 g
- Sugar: 10 g

Cooking time: 40 minutes

Recipe 3:

Black Bean and Sweet Potato Enchiladas

Ingredients:
- 1 tablespoon of coconut oil
- 1 onion, chopped
- 3 cloves of garlic, minced
- 2 teaspoons of chili powder
- 1 teaspoon of cumin
- 1/4 teaspoon of smoked paprika
- Salt and pepper, to taste
- 2 cups of cooked black beans
- 2 cups of mashed sweet potatoes
- 12 gluten-free tortillas
- 2 cups of enchilada sauce
- 1/4 cup of vegan cheese shreds (optional)
- 2 tablespoons of chopped cilantro

Preparation:
- Preheat the oven to 180°C (350°F) and grease a 9x13 inch baking dish.
- In a large skillet over medium-high heat, heat the coconut oil and sauté the onion, garlic, chili powder, cumin, smoked paprika, salt, and pepper for 10 minutes, until soft and fragrant.

- In a medium bowl, mash the black beans with a fork or a potato masher. Stir in the sweet potatoes and mix well.
- To assemble the enchiladas, spoon about 1/4 cup of the bean and sweet potato mixture on each tortilla. Roll up tightly and place seam-side down in the prepared baking dish. Pour the enchilada sauce over the top and sprinkle with vegan cheese if using.
- Bake for 25 to 30 minutes, until the sauce is bubbly and the cheese is melted.
- Sprinkle with cilantro and enjoy a spicy and filling dinner.

Nutritional value (per serving):
- Calories: 320 kcal
- Protein: 10 g
- Fat: 8 g
- Carbohydrates: 54 g
- Fiber: 11 g
- Sugar: 9 g

Cooking time: 50 minutes

Recipe 4:

Creamy Mushroom and Spinach Pasta

Ingredients:
- 8 ounces of gluten-free pasta of choice
- 2 tablespoons of olive oil
- 4 cups of mushrooms, sliced
- Salt and pepper, to taste
- 2 tablespoons of gluten-free all-purpose flour
- 2 cups of unsweetened almond milk
- 2 teaspoons of dried parsley
- 2 teaspoons of dried basil
- 1/4 teaspoon of nutmeg
- 4 cups of baby spinach
- 1/4 cup of nutritional yeast

Preparation:
- Cook the pasta according to the package directions, until al dente. Drain and set aside.
- In a large skillet over medium-high heat, heat the olive oil and sauté the mushrooms with salt and pepper for 15 minutes, until browned and tender.
- Sprinkle the flour over the mushrooms and stir to coat. Gradually whisk in the almond milk, stirring constantly to avoid lumps.

Bring the sauce to a boil, then reduce the heat and simmer, stirring occasionally, for 10 minutes, until thickened.

- Stir in the parsley, basil, nutmeg, spinach, and nutritional yeast. Cook for another 5 minutes, until the spinach is wilted.

- Add the pasta to the skillet and toss to combine. Enjoy a creamy and satisfying dinner.

Nutritional value (per serving):
- Calories: 360 kcal
- Protein: 14 g
- Fat: 11 g
- Carbohydrates: 55 g
- Fiber: 9 g
- Sugar: 8 g

Cooking time: 35 minutes

Recipe 5:

Vegetable and Tofu Stir-Fry with Brown Rice

Ingredients:

- 2 cups of cooked brown rice
- 1/4 cup of gluten-free soy sauce or tamari
- 2 tablespoons of rice vinegar
- 2 tablespoons of maple syrup
- 1 tablespoon of cornstarch
- 1 teaspoon of sesame oil
- 1/4 teaspoon of red pepper flakes
- 1 tablespoon of coconut oil
- 1 14-ounce block of extra-firm tofu, drained, pressed, and cubed
- Salt and pepper, to taste
- 2 cups of broccoli florets
- 2 cups of snow peas
- 2 carrots, peeled and sliced
- 2 green onions, sliced
- 2 teaspoons of sesame seeds

Preparation:
- In a small bowl, whisk together the soy sauce or tamari, rice vinegar, maple syrup, cornstarch, sesame oil, and red pepper flakes. Set aside.
- In a large skillet over medium-high heat, heat the coconut oil and fry the tofu for 15 to 20 minutes, turning occasionally, until golden and crisp. Season with salt and pepper and transfer to a plate.
- In the same skillet over medium-high heat, add the broccoli, snow peas, and carrots and stir-fry for 10 minutes, until crisp-tender. Add the sauce and bring to a boil.

Reduce the heat and simmer, stirring occasionally, for 5 minutes, until the sauce is thickened.
- Stir in the tofu and heat through.
- Serve over brown rice and garnish with green onions and sesame seeds. Enjoy a colorful and tasty dinner.

Nutritional value (per serving):
- Calories: 400 kcal
- Protein: 18 g
- Fat: 14 g
- Carbohydrates: 56 g
- Fiber: 8 g
- Sugar: 16 g

Cooking time: 45 minutes

Recipe 6:

Vegetable and Bean Chili with Cornbread

Ingredients:
- 1 tablespoon of olive oil
- 1 onion, chopped
- 3 cloves of garlic, minced

- 1 green bell pepper, chopped
- 1 red bell pepper, chopped
- 2 tablespoons of chili powder
- 1 teaspoon of cumin
- 1/4 teaspoon of smoked paprika
- Salt and pepper, to taste
- 1 28-ounce can of diced tomatoes
- 1 15-ounce can of black beans, drained and rinsed
- 1 15-ounce can of kidney beans, drained and rinsed
- 1 15-ounce can of corn, drained
- 1/4 cup of chopped cilantro
- 1 batch of gluten-free cornbread (see [recipe](^1^))

Preparation:

- In a large pot over medium-high heat, heat the olive oil and sauté the onion, garlic, bell peppers, chili powder, cumin, smoked paprika, salt, and pepper for 10 minutes, until soft and fragrant.
- Add the tomatoes, beans, and corn and bring to a boil. Reduce the heat and simmer, uncovered, for 20 minutes, until the chili is thick and hearty.
- Stir in the cilantro and serve with cornbread. Enjoy a warm and spicy dinner.

Nutritional value (per serving):

- Calories: 360 kcal
- Protein: 15 g
- Fat: 8 g
- Carbohydrates: 60 g
- Fiber: 15 g
- Sugar: 15 g

Cooking time: 40 minutes

Recipe 7:

Roasted Vegetable and Quinoa Buddha Bowl

Ingredients:
- 2 cups of cooked quinoa
- 2 cups of broccoli florets
- 2 cups of cauliflower florets
- 2 cups of Brussels sprouts, halved
- 2 tablespoons of olive oil
- Salt and pepper, to taste
- 1/4 cup of tahini
- 2 tablespoons of lemon juice
- 2 tablespoons of water
- 1 teaspoon of maple syrup
- 1/4 teaspoon of garlic powder

- 1/4 teaspoon of cumin
- 4 cups of baby spinach
- 1/4 cup of pumpkin seeds

Preparation:
- Preheat the oven to 200°C (400°F) and line two baking sheets with parchment paper.
- In a large bowl, toss the broccoli, cauliflower, and Brussels sprouts with the olive oil, salt, and pepper. Spread them on the prepared baking sheets in a single layer. Roast for 25 to 30 minutes, until tender and browned, flipping halfway through.
- In a small bowl, whisk together the tahini, lemon juice, water, maple syrup, garlic powder, and cumin. Adjust the consistency and seasoning as needed.
- To serve, divide the quinoa among four bowls and top with spinach, roasted vegetables, and pumpkin seeds. Drizzle with the tahini dressing and enjoy a nutritious and satisfying dinner.

Nutritional value (per serving):
- Calories: 420 kcal
- Protein: 16 g
- Fat: 22 g
- Carbohydrates: 46 g
- Fiber: 12 g
- Sugar: 10 g

Cooking time: 40 minutes

Recipe 8:

Black Bean and Sweet Potato Enchiladas

Ingredients:
- 1 tablespoon of coconut oil
- 1 onion, chopped
- 3 cloves of garlic, minced
- 2 teaspoons of chili powder
- 1 teaspoon of cumin
- 1/4 teaspoon of smoked paprika
- Salt and pepper, to taste
- 2 cups of cooked black beans
- 2 cups of mashed sweet potatoes
- 12 gluten-free tortillas
- 2 cups of enchilada sauce
- 1/4 cup of vegan cheese shreds (optional)
- 2 tablespoons of chopped cilantro

Preparation:
- Preheat the oven to 180°C (350°F) and grease a 9x13 inch baking dish.
- In a large skillet over medium-high heat, heat the coconut oil and sauté the onion, garlic, chili powder, cumin, smoked paprika, salt, and pepper for 10 minutes, until soft and fragrant.

- In a medium bowl, mash the black beans with a fork or a potato masher. Stir in the sweet potatoes and mix well.

- To assemble the enchiladas, spoon about 1/4 cup of the bean and sweet potato mixture on each tortilla. Roll up tightly and place seam-side down in the prepared baking dish. Pour the enchilada sauce over the top and sprinkle with vegan cheese if using.

- Bake for 25 to 30 minutes, until the sauce is bubbly and the cheese is melted.

- Sprinkle with cilantro and enjoy a spicy and filling dinner.

Nutritional value (per serving):
- Calories: 320 kcal
- Protein: 10 g
- Fat: 8 g
- Carbohydrates: 54 g
- Fiber: 11 g
- Sugar: 9 g

Cooking time: 50 minutes

Recipe 9:

Creamy Mushroom and Spinach Pasta

Ingredients:
- 8 ounces of gluten-free pasta of choice
- 2 tablespoons of olive oil
- 4 cups of mushrooms, sliced
- Salt and pepper, to taste
- 2 tablespoons of gluten-free all-purpose flour
- 2 cups of unsweetened almond milk
- 2 teaspoons of dried parsley
- 2 teaspoons of dried basil
- 1/4 teaspoon of nutmeg
- 4 cups of baby spinach
- 1/4 cup of nutritional yeast

Preparation:
- Cook the pasta according to the package directions, until al dente. Drain and set aside.
- In a large skillet over medium-high heat, heat the olive oil and sauté the mushrooms with salt and pepper for 15 minutes, until browned and tender.
- Sprinkle the flour over the mushrooms and stir to coat. Gradually whisk in the almond milk, stirring constantly to avoid lumps.

Bring the sauce to a boil, then reduce the heat and simmer, stirring occasionally, for 10 minutes, until thickened.

- Stir in the parsley, basil, nutmeg, spinach, and nutritional yeast. Cook for another 5 minutes, until the spinach is wilted.

- Add the pasta to the skillet and toss to combine. Enjoy a creamy and satisfying dinner.

Nutritional value (per serving):
- Calories: 360 kcal
- Protein: 14 g
- Fat: 11 g
- Carbohydrates: 55 g
- Fiber: 9 g
- Sugar: 8 g

Cooking time: 35 minutes

Recipe 10:

Vegetable and Tofu Stir-Fry with Brown Rice

Ingredients:

- 2 cups of cooked brown rice
- 1/4 cup of gluten-free soy sauce or tamari
- 2 tablespoons of rice vinegar
- 2 tablespoons of maple syrup
- 1 tablespoon of cornstarch
- 1 teaspoon of sesame oil
- 1/4 teaspoon of red pepper flakes
- 1 tablespoon of coconut oil
- 1 14-ounce block of extra-firm tofu, drained, pressed, and cubed
- Salt and pepper, to taste
- 2 cups of broccoli florets
- 2 cups of snow peas
- 2 carrots, peeled and sliced
- 2 green onions, sliced
- 2 teaspoons of sesame seeds

Preparation:

- In a small bowl, whisk together the soy sauce or tamari, rice vinegar, maple syrup, cornstarch, sesame oil, and red pepper flakes. Set aside.
- In a large skillet over medium-high heat, heat the coconut oil and fry the tofu for 15 to 20 minutes, turning occasionally, until golden and crisp. Season with salt and pepper and transfer to a plate.
- In the same skillet over medium-high heat, add the broccoli, snow peas, and carrots and stir-fry for 10 minutes, until crisp-tender. Add the sauce and bring to a boil.

Reduce the heat and simmer, stirring occasionally, for 5 minutes, until the sauce is thickened.
- Stir in the tofu and heat through.
- Serve over brown rice and garnish with green onions and sesame seeds. Enjoy a colorful and tasty dinner.

Nutritional value (per serving):
- Calories: 400 kcal
- Protein: 18 g
- Fat: 14 g
- Carbohydrates: 56 g
- Fiber: 8 g
- Sugar: 16 g

Cooking time: 45 minutes

Chapter 5:

Decadent Desserts

Recipe 1:

Strawberry and Coconut Ice Cream

Ingredients:
- 2 cups of frozen strawberries
- 1 cup of full-fat coconut milk
- 2 tablespoons of maple syrup
- 1 teaspoon of vanilla extract

Preparation:
- In a blender, combine the strawberries, coconut milk, maple syrup, and vanilla. Blend until smooth and creamy.
- Transfer the mixture to a freezer-safe container and freeze for at least 4 hours, or until firm.
- Enjoy as a refreshing and fruity ice cream.

Nutritional value (per serving):
- Calories: 200 kcal
- Protein: 2 g
- Fat: 14 g

- Carbohydrates: 18 g
- Fiber: 3 g
- Sugar: 14 g

Cooking time: 10 minutes (plus freezing time)

Recipe 2:

Cinnamon and Raisin Bread Pudding

Ingredients:
- 4 slices of gluten-free bread, cubed
- 2 cups of unsweetened almond milk
- 2 tablespoons of maple syrup
- 2 teaspoons of vanilla extract
- 1 teaspoon of cinnamon
- 1/4 teaspoon of nutmeg
- 1/4 cup of raisins
- 2 tablespoons of chopped walnuts

Preparation:
- Preheat the oven to 180°C (350°F) and grease a baking dish.
- In a large bowl, whisk together the almond milk, maple syrup, vanilla, cinnamon, and nutmeg.

- Add the bread cubes and raisins and toss to coat well.
- Transfer the mixture to the prepared baking dish and sprinkle with walnuts.
- Bake for 25 to 30 minutes, until golden and set.
- Enjoy as a warm and cozy dessert.

Nutritional value (per serving):
- Calories: 260 kcal
- Protein: 6 g
- Fat: 9 g
- Carbohydrates: 41 g
- Fiber: 4 g
- Sugar: 19 g

Cooking time: 40 minutes

Recipe 3:

Quick and Easy Strawberry Tart

Ingredients:
- 1 1/2 cups of almond flour
- 1/4 cup of coconut oil, melted
- 2 tablespoons of maple syrup
- A pinch of salt
- 1/4 cup of coconut cream

- 2 tablespoons of powdered erythritol
- 1 teaspoon of vanilla extract
- 2 cups of fresh strawberries, sliced

Preparation:
- Preheat the oven to 180°C (350°F) and line a tart pan with parchment paper.
- In a medium bowl, mix together the almond flour, coconut oil, maple syrup, and salt. Press the dough evenly into the bottom and sides of the prepared tart pan. Prick the dough with a fork and bake for 15 minutes, until golden and firm.
- In a small bowl, whisk together the coconut cream, erythritol, and vanilla. Spread the cream over the crust and arrange the strawberry slices on top.
- Refrigerate the tart for at least 2 hours, or until set.
- Enjoy as a simple and elegant dessert.

Nutritional value (per serving):
- Calories: 280 kcal
- Protein: 6 g
- Fat: 23 g
- Carbohydrates: 16 g
- Fiber: 4 g
- Sugar: 10 g

Cooking time: 25 minutes (plus refrigeration time)

Recipe 4: Buckwheat Berry Pie

Ingredients:
- 1 cup of buckwheat flour
- 1/4 cup of coconut oil, melted
- 2 tablespoons of maple syrup
- A pinch of salt
- 2 cups of mixed berries, fresh or frozen
- 2 tablespoons of cornstarch
- 2 tablespoons of water
- 2 tablespoons of lemon juice
- 2 tablespoons of coconut sugar

Preparation:
- Preheat the oven to 180°C (350°F) and grease a pie dish.
- In a medium bowl, mix together the buckwheat flour, coconut oil, maple syrup, and salt. Press the dough evenly into the bottom and sides of the prepared pie dish. Prick the dough with a fork and bake for 15 minutes, until golden and firm.
- In a small saucepan, combine the berries, cornstarch, water, lemon juice, and coconut sugar. Bring to a boil, then reduce the heat and simmer, stirring occasionally, for 10 minutes, until the berries are soft and the sauce is thickened.
- Pour the berry mixture over the crust and spread evenly.

- Bake for another 10 minutes, until bubbly.
- Let the pie cool slightly before slicing and serving.
- Enjoy as a fruity and gluten-free dessert.

Nutritional value (per serving):
- Calories: 250 kcal
- Protein: 3 g
- Fat: 12 g
- Carbohydrates: 36 g
- Fiber: 5 g
- Sugar: 18 g

Cooking time: 40 minutes

Recipe 5:

Chia Pudding with Coconut Milk, Mango, and Coconut Flakes

Ingredients:
- 1/4 cup of chia seeds
- 1 cup of coconut milk
- 2 tablespoons of maple syrup
- 1/4 teaspoon of vanilla extract
- 1/4 teaspoon of cardamom
- 1 cup of diced mango, fresh or frozen

- 2 tablespoons of coconut flakes, toasted

Preparation:
- In a small bowl, whisk together the chia seeds, coconut milk, maple syrup, vanilla, and cardamom. Refrigerate for at least 4 hours, or overnight, until thick and gel-like.
- In a small skillet over medium heat, toast the coconut flakes, stirring frequently, until golden and crisp, about 5 minutes. Transfer to a plate and let cool.
- To serve, divide the chia pudding among two bowls and top with mango and coconut flakes.
- Enjoy as a tropical and creamy dessert.

Nutritional value (per serving):
- Calories: 400 kcal
- Protein: 7 g
- Fat: 27 g
- Carbohydrates: 39 g
- Fiber: 13 g
- Sugar: 25 g

Cooking time: 10 minutes (plus refrigeration time)

Recipe 6:

Chocolate Avocado Pudding

Ingredients:
- 2 ripe avocados, peeled and pitted
- 1/4 cup of unsweetened cocoa powder
- 1/4 cup of maple syrup
- 1/4 cup of almond milk
- 1 teaspoon of vanilla extract
- A pinch of salt
- Fresh berries, for topping (optional)

Preparation:
- In a blender or food processor, combine the avocados, cocoa powder, maple syrup, almond milk, vanilla, and salt. Blend until smooth and creamy, scraping down the sides as needed.
- Transfer the pudding to a bowl and refrigerate for at least an hour, or until chilled.
- Serve with fresh berries if desired. Enjoy as a rich and decadent dessert.

Nutritional value (per serving):
- Calories: 280 kcal
- Protein: 4 g
- Fat: 18 g
- Carbohydrates: 32 g

- Fiber: 10 g
- Sugar: 18 g

Cooking time: 10 minutes (plus chilling time)

Recipe 7:

Coconut Rice Pudding with Mango

Ingredients:
- 1 cup of uncooked white rice
- 2 cups of water
- 2 cups of coconut milk
- 1/4 cup of coconut sugar
- 1/4 teaspoon of cardamom
- 1/4 teaspoon of cinnamon
- A pinch of salt
- 1 ripe mango, peeled and diced
- 2 tablespoons of shredded coconut, toasted

Preparation:
- In a medium saucepan, bring the rice and water to a boil. Reduce the heat and simmer, covered, for 15 to 20 minutes, until the rice is tender and the water is absorbed.
- Stir in the coconut milk, coconut sugar, cardamom, cinnamon, and salt.

Bring the mixture to a boil, then reduce the heat and simmer, uncovered, for 20 to 25 minutes, stirring occasionally, until the pudding is thick and creamy.
- Serve the pudding warm or cold, topped with mango and shredded coconut. Enjoy as a tropical and comforting dessert.

Nutritional value (per serving):
- Calories: 360 kcal
- Protein: 5 g
- Fat: 18 g
- Carbohydrates: 48 g
- Fiber: 3 g
- Sugar: 20 g

Cooking time: 50 minutes

Recipe 8:

Banana and Peanut Butter Oat Bars

Ingredients:
- 2 ripe bananas, mashed
- 1/4 cup of natural peanut butter
- 2 tablespoons of maple syrup
- 1 teaspoon of vanilla extract
- 2 cups of gluten-free rolled oats

- 1/4 cup of chopped peanuts
- 1/4 cup of dairy-free chocolate chips

Preparation:

- Preheat the oven to 180°C (350°F) and line an 8x8 inch baking pan with parchment paper.
- In a large bowl, whisk together the bananas, peanut butter, maple syrup, and vanilla. Stir in the oats, peanuts, and chocolate chips and mix well.
- Press the mixture evenly into the prepared baking pan and bake for 25 to 30 minutes, until golden and firm.
- Let the bars cool completely in the pan before cutting into 16 squares. Enjoy as a chewy and satisfying dessert.

Nutritional value (per serving):

- Calories: 140 kcal
- Protein: 4 g
- Fat: 6 g
- Carbohydrates: 19 g
- Fiber: 3 g
- Sugar: 8 g

Cooking time: 40 minutes

Recipe 9:

Lemon and Poppy Seed Cake

Ingredients:
- 2 cups of almond flour
- 1/4 cup of coconut flour
- 1/4 cup of poppy seeds
- 2 teaspoons of baking powder
- A pinch of salt
- 1/2 cup of coconut oil, melted
- 1/2 cup of maple syrup
- 1/4 cup of lemon juice
- 2 teaspoons of lemon zest
- 2 flax eggs (2 tablespoons of ground flax seeds mixed with 6 tablespoons of water)

Preparation:
- Preheat the oven to 180°C (350°F) and grease a loaf pan.
- In a large bowl, whisk together the almond flour, coconut flour, poppy seeds, baking powder, and salt.
- In a small bowl, whisk together the coconut oil, maple syrup, lemon juice, lemon zest, and flax eggs.
- Add the wet ingredients to the dry ingredients and stir to combine. Pour the batter into the prepared loaf pan and smooth the top.

- Bake for 35 to 40 minutes, until a toothpick inserted in the center comes out clean.
- Let the cake cool slightly in the pan before transferring to a wire rack to cool completely.
- Enjoy as a zesty and moist dessert.

Nutritional value (per serving):
- Calories: 280 kcal
- Protein: 7 g
- Fat: 21 g
- Carbohydrates: 19 g
- Fiber: 5 g
- Sugar: 11 g

Cooking time: 50 minutes

Recipe 10:

Apple and Cinnamon Crisp

Ingredients:
- 4 large apples, peeled, cored, and sliced
- 2 tablespoons of lemon juice
- 2 tablespoons of coconut sugar
- 1 teaspoon of cinnamon
- 1/4 teaspoon of nutmeg
- 1 cup of gluten-free rolled oats

- 1/4 cup of almond flour
- 1/4 cup of coconut oil, melted
- 2 tablespoons of maple syrup
- A pinch of salt

Preparation:
- Preheat the oven to 180°C (350°F) and grease an 8x8 inch baking dish.
- In a large bowl, toss the apple slices with the lemon juice, coconut sugar, cinnamon, and nutmeg. Transfer the apple mixture to the prepared baking dish and spread it evenly.
- In a small bowl, stir together the oats, almond flour, coconut oil, maple syrup, and salt. Sprinkle the oat mixture over the apple layer and press lightly.
- Bake for 30 to 35 minutes, until the topping is golden and the apples are bubbly.
- Enjoy as a warm and cozy dessert.

Nutritional value (per serving):
- Calories: 260 kcal
- Protein: 3 g
- Fat: 14 g
- Carbohydrates: 34 g
- Fiber: 5 g
- Sugar: 20 g

Cooking time: 45 minutes

Chapter 6:

Snacks and Small Bites

Recipe 1:

Chocolate Avocado Pudding

Ingredients:
- 2 ripe avocados, peeled and pitted
- 1/4 cup of unsweetened cocoa powder
- 1/4 cup of maple syrup
- 1/4 cup of almond milk
- 1 teaspoon of vanilla extract
- A pinch of salt
- Fresh berries, for topping (optional)

Preparation:
- In a blender or food processor, combine the avocados, cocoa powder, maple syrup, almond milk, vanilla, and salt. Blend until smooth and creamy, scraping down the sides as needed.

- Transfer the pudding to a bowl and refrigerate for at least an hour, or until chilled.
- Serve with fresh berries if desired. Enjoy as a rich and decadent snack.

Nutritional value (per serving):
- Calories: 280 kcal
- Protein: 4 g
- Fat: 18 g
- Carbohydrates: 32 g
- Fiber: 10 g
- Sugar: 18 g

Cooking time: 10 minutes (plus chilling time)

Recipe 2:

Coconut Rice Pudding with Mango

Ingredients:
- 1 cup of uncooked white rice
- 2 cups of water
- 2 cups of coconut milk
- 1/4 cup of coconut sugar
- 1/4 teaspoon of cardamom
- 1/4 teaspoon of cinnamon
- A pinch of salt

- 1 ripe mango, peeled and diced
- 2 tablespoons of shredded coconut, toasted

Preparation:
- In a medium saucepan, bring the rice and water to a boil. Reduce the heat and simmer, covered, for 15 to 20 minutes, until the rice is tender and the water is absorbed.
- Stir in the coconut milk, coconut sugar, cardamom, cinnamon, and salt. Bring the mixture to a boil, then reduce the heat and simmer, uncovered, for 20 to 25 minutes, stirring occasionally, until the pudding is thick and creamy.
- Serve the pudding warm or cold, topped with mango and shredded coconut. Enjoy as a tropical and comforting snack.

Nutritional value (per serving):
- Calories: 360 kcal
- Protein: 5 g
- Fat: 18 g
- Carbohydrates: 48 g
- Fiber: 3 g
- Sugar: 20 g

Cooking time: 50 minutes

Recipe 3:

Banana and Peanut Butter Oat Bars

Ingredients:
- 2 ripe bananas, mashed
- 1/4 cup of natural peanut butter
- 2 tablespoons of maple syrup
- 1 teaspoon of vanilla extract
- 2 cups of gluten-free rolled oats
- 1/4 cup of chopped peanuts
- 1/4 cup of dairy-free chocolate chips

Preparation:
- Preheat the oven to 180°C (350°F) and line an 8x8 inch baking pan with parchment paper.
- In a large bowl, whisk together the bananas, peanut butter, maple syrup, and vanilla. Stir in the oats, peanuts, and chocolate chips and mix well.
- Press the mixture evenly into the prepared baking pan and bake for 25 to 30 minutes, until golden and firm.
- Let the bars cool completely in the pan before cutting into 16 squares. Enjoy as a chewy and satisfying snack.

Nutritional value (per serving):
- Calories: 140 kcal
- Protein: 4 g
- Fat: 6 g
- Carbohydrates: 19 g
- Fiber: 3 g
- Sugar: 8 g

Cooking time: 40 minutes

Recipe 4:

Lemon and Poppy Seed Cake

Ingredients:
- 2 cups of almond flour
- 1/4 cup of coconut flour
- 1/4 cup of poppy seeds
- 2 teaspoons of baking powder
- A pinch of salt
- 1/2 cup of coconut oil, melted
- 1/2 cup of maple syrup
- 1/4 cup of lemon juice
- 2 teaspoons of lemon zest
- 2 flax eggs (2 tablespoons of ground flax seeds mixed with 6 tablespoons of water)

Preparation:
- Preheat the oven to 180°C (350°F) and grease a loaf pan.
- In a large bowl, whisk together the almond flour, coconut flour, poppy seeds, baking powder, and salt.
- In a small bowl, whisk together the coconut oil, maple syrup, lemon juice, lemon zest, and flax eggs.
- Add the wet ingredients to the dry ingredients and stir to combine. Pour the batter into the prepared loaf pan and smooth the top.
- Bake for 35 to 40 minutes, until a toothpick inserted in the center comes out clean.
- Let the cake cool slightly in the pan before transferring to a wire rack to cool completely.
- Enjoy as a zesty and moist snack.

Nutritional value (per serving):
- Calories: 280 kcal
- Protein: 7 g
- Fat: 21 g
- Carbohydrates: 19 g
- Fiber: 5 g
- Sugar: 11 g

Cooking time: 50 minutes

Recipe 5:

Apple and Cinnamon Crisp

Ingredients:
- 4 large apples, peeled, cored, and sliced
- 2 tablespoons of lemon juice
- 2 tablespoons of coconut sugar
- 1 teaspoon of cinnamon
- 1/4 teaspoon of nutmeg
- 1 cup of gluten-free rolled oats
- 1/4 cup of almond flour
- 1/4 cup of coconut oil, melted
- 2 tablespoons of maple syrup
- A pinch of salt

Preparation:
- Preheat the oven to 180°C (350°F) and grease an 8x8 inch baking dish.
- In a large bowl, toss the apple slices with the lemon juice, coconut sugar, cinnamon, and nutmeg. Transfer the apple mixture to the prepared baking dish and spread it evenly.
- In a small bowl, stir together the oats, almond flour, coconut oil, maple syrup, and salt. Sprinkle the oat mixture over the apple layer and press lightly.

- Bake for 30 to 35 minutes, until the topping is golden and the apples are bubbly.
- Enjoy as a warm and cozy snack.

Nutritional value (per serving):
- Calories: 260 kcal
- Protein: 3 g
- Fat: 14 g
- Carbohydrates: 34 g
- Fiber: 5 g
- Sugar: 20 g

Cooking time: 45 minutes

Recipe 6:

Chocolate Avocado Pudding

Ingredients:
- 2 ripe avocados, peeled and pitted
- 1/4 cup of unsweetened cocoa powder
- 1/4 cup of maple syrup
- 1/4 cup of almond milk
- 1 teaspoon of vanilla extract
- A pinch of salt
- Fresh berries, for topping (optional)

Preparation:

- In a blender or food processor, combine the avocados, cocoa powder, maple syrup, almond milk, vanilla, and salt. Blend until smooth and creamy, scraping down the sides as needed.
- Transfer the pudding to a bowl and refrigerate for at least an hour, or until chilled.
- Serve with fresh berries if desired. Enjoy as a rich and decadent snack.

Nutritional value (per serving):
- Calories: 280 kcal
- Protein: 4 g
- Fat: 18 g
- Carbohydrates: 32 g
- Fiber: 10 g
- Sugar: 18 g

Cooking time: 10 minutes (plus chilling time)

Recipe 7:

Coconut Rice Pudding with Mango

Ingredients:

- 1 cup of uncooked white rice
- 2 cups of water
- 2 cups of coconut milk
- 1/4 cup of coconut sugar
- 1/4 teaspoon of cardamom
- 1/4 teaspoon of cinnamon
- A pinch of salt
- 1 ripe mango, peeled and diced
- 2 tablespoons of shredded coconut, toasted

Preparation:

- In a medium saucepan, bring the rice and water to a boil. Reduce the heat and simmer, covered, for 15 to 20 minutes, until the rice is tender and the water is absorbed.

- Stir in the coconut milk, coconut sugar, cardamom, cinnamon, and salt. Bring the mixture to a boil, then reduce the heat and simmer, uncovered, for 20 to 25 minutes, stirring occasionally, until the pudding is thick and creamy.

- Serve the pudding warm or cold, topped with mango and shredded coconut. Enjoy as a tropical and comforting snack.

Nutritional value (per serving):
- Calories: 360 kcal
- Protein: 5 g
- Fat: 18 g
- Carbohydrates: 48 g

- Fiber: 3 g
- Sugar: 20 g

Cooking time: 50 minutes

Recipe 8:

Banana and Peanut Butter Oat Bars

Ingredients:
- 2 ripe bananas, mashed
- 1/4 cup of natural peanut butter
- 2 tablespoons of maple syrup
- 1 teaspoon of vanilla extract
- 2 cups of gluten-free rolled oats
- 1/4 cup of chopped peanuts
- 1/4 cup of dairy-free chocolate chips

Preparation:
- Preheat the oven to 180°C (350°F) and line an 8x8 inch baking pan with parchment paper.
- In a large bowl, whisk together the bananas, peanut butter, maple syrup, and vanilla. Stir in the oats, peanuts, and chocolate chips and mix well.
- Press the mixture evenly into the prepared baking pan and bake for 25 to 30 minutes, until golden and firm.

- Let the bars cool completely in the pan before cutting into 16 squares. Enjoy as a chewy and satisfying snack.

Nutritional value (per serving):
- Calories: 140 kcal
- Protein: 4 g
- Fat: 6 g
- Carbohydrates: 19 g
- Fiber: 3 g
- Sugar: 8 g

Cooking time: 40 minutes

Recipe 9:

Lemon and Poppy Seed Cake

Ingredients:
- 2 cups of almond flour
- 1/4 cup of coconut flour
- 1/4 cup of poppy seeds
- 2 teaspoons of baking powder
- A pinch of salt
- 1/2 cup of coconut oil, melted
- 1/2 cup of maple syrup
- 1/4 cup of lemon juice

- 2 teaspoons of lemon zest
- 2 flax eggs (2 tablespoons of ground flax seeds mixed with 6 tablespoons of water)

Preparation:
- Preheat the oven to 180°C (350°F) and grease a loaf pan.
- In a large bowl, whisk together the almond flour, coconut flour, poppy seeds, baking powder, and salt.
- In a small bowl, whisk together the coconut oil, maple syrup, lemon juice, lemon zest, and flax eggs.
- Add the wet ingredients to the dry ingredients and stir to combine. Pour the batter into the prepared loaf pan and smooth the top.
- Bake for 35 to 40 minutes, until a toothpick inserted in the center comes out clean.
- Let the cake cool slightly in the pan before transferring to a wire rack to cool completely.
- Enjoy as a zesty and moist snack.

Nutritional value (per serving):
- Calories: 280 kcal
- Protein: 7 g
- Fat: 21 g
- Carbohydrates: 19 g
- Fiber: 5 g
- Sugar: 11 g

Cooking time: 50 minutes

Recipe 10:

Apple and Cinnamon Crisp

Ingredients:
- 4 large apples, peeled, cored, and sliced
- 2 tablespoons of lemon juice
- 2 tablespoons of coconut sugar
- 1 teaspoon of cinnamon
- 1/4 teaspoon of nutmeg
- 1 cup of gluten-free rolled oats
- 1/4 cup of almond flour
- 1/4 cup of coconut oil, melted
- 2 tablespoons of maple syrup
- A pinch of salt

Preparation:
- Preheat the oven to 180°C (350°F) and grease an 8x8 inch baking dish.
- In a large bowl, toss the apple slices with the lemon juice, coconut sugar, cinnamon, and nutmeg. Transfer the apple mixture to the prepared baking dish and spread it evenly.
- In a small bowl, stir together the oats, almond flour, coconut oil, maple syrup, and salt. Sprinkle the oat mixture over the apple layer and press lightly.

- Bake for 30 to 35 minutes, until the topping is golden and the apples are bubbly.
- Enjoy as a warm and cozy snack.

Nutritional value (per serving):
- Calories: 260 kcal
- Protein: 3 g
- Fat: 14 g
- Carbohydrates: 34 g
- Fiber: 5 g
- Sugar: 20 g

Cooking time: 45 minutes

Chapter 7:

Beverages and Refreshments

Recipe 1:

Anti-Inflammatory Blueberry Hemp Seed Smoothie

Ingredients:
- 1 1/4 cup (140 g) frozen blueberries (or other frozen berry of choice)
- 2 tbsp (22 g) hemp seeds
- 1 serving (30 g) vanilla plant-based protein powder
- 1/2 cup packed (30 g), fresh spinach or kale
- 1 tsp spirulina or chlorella powder
- 1 1/4 unsweetened plant-based milk of choice
- 1/4 tsp holy basil powder (optional)

Preparation:

- In a blender, combine all the ingredients and blend until smooth and creamy.
- Enjoy as a refreshing and anti-inflammatory smoothie.

Nutritional value (per serving):
- Calories: 320 kcal
- Protein: 24 g
- Fat: 14 g
- Carbohydrates: 32 g
- Fiber: 8 g
- Sugar: 18 g

Cooking time: 5 minutes

Recipe 2:

Superfoods Detox Smoothie

Ingredients:
- 2 cups freshly squeezed orange juice, or equal quantity peeled and pitted oranges
- 1 unpeeled, pitted apple
- 1 ripe banana
- 3 tablespoons goji berries

- 1 teaspoon turmeric
- A pinch of pepper
- 1 teaspoon cinnamon
- 2 tablespoons tahini (you can up this to 4 tablespoons or even replace with almond butter)
- 3 brazil nuts
- 2 teaspoons fresh grated ginger
- 3 teaspoons chia seeds

Preparation:
- In a blender, combine all the ingredients and blend until smooth and frothy.
- Enjoy as a detoxifying and energizing smoothie.

Nutritional value (per serving):
- Calories: 420 kcal
- Protein: 10 g
- Fat: 18 g
- Carbohydrates: 60 g
- Fiber: 12 g
- Sugar: 36 g

Cooking time: 10 minutes

Recipe 3:

Coconut and Turmeric Latte

Ingredients:
- 1 cup of coconut milk
- 1/2 teaspoon of turmeric
- 1/4 teaspoon of cinnamon
- A pinch of black pepper
- 1 teaspoon of maple syrup
- 1/4 teaspoon of vanilla extract

Preparation:
- In a small saucepan over medium heat, whisk together the coconut milk, turmeric, cinnamon, pepper, maple syrup, and vanilla. Bring to a boil, then reduce the heat and simmer for 5 minutes, stirring occasionally.
- Enjoy as a warm and anti-inflammatory latte.

Nutritional value (per serving):
- Calories: 240 kcal
- Protein: 2 g
- Fat: 22 g
- Carbohydrates: 12 g
- Fiber: 2 g
- Sugar: 8 g

Cooking time: 10 minutes

Recipe 4:

Cacao and Maca Smoothie

Ingredients:
- 1 cup of almond milk
- 1 ripe banana
- 2 tablespoons of raw cacao powder
- 1 tablespoon of maca powder
- 1 tablespoon of almond butter
- 1 teaspoon of maple syrup
- A pinch of salt

Preparation:
- In a blender, combine all the ingredients and blend until smooth and creamy.
- Enjoy as a chocolatey and hormone-balancing smoothie.

Nutritional value (per serving):
- Calories: 360 kcal
- Protein: 10 g
- Fat: 18 g
- Carbohydrates: 46 g
- Fiber: 10 g

- Sugar: 24 g

Cooking time: 5 minutes

Recipe 5:

Ginger and Lemon Tea

Ingredients:
- 4 cups of water
- 2 inches of fresh ginger, peeled and sliced
- 1/4 cup of fresh lemon juice
- 2 tablespoons of honey
- A pinch of cayenne pepper (optional)

Preparation:
- In a medium saucepan over high heat, bring the water and ginger to a boil. Reduce the heat and simmer for 15 minutes, until the ginger is infused.
- Strain the tea and stir in the lemon juice, honey, and cayenne if using.
- Enjoy as a soothing and immune-boosting tea.

Nutritional value (per serving):
- Calories: 60 kcal
- Protein: 0 g
- Fat: 0 g

- Carbohydrates: 18 g
- Fiber: 0 g
- Sugar: 16 g

Cooking time: 20 minutes

Recipe 6:

Anti-Inflammatory Blueberry Hemp Seed Smoothie

Ingredients:

- 1 1/4 cup (140 g) frozen blueberries (or other frozen berry of choice)
- 2 tbsp (22 g) hemp seeds
- 1 serving (30 g) vanilla plant-based protein powder
- 1/2 cup packed (30 g), fresh spinach or kale
- 1 tsp spirulina or chlorella powder
- 1 1/4 unsweetened plant-based milk of choice
- 1/4 tsp holy basil powder (optional)

Preparation:

- In a blender, combine all the ingredients and blend until smooth and creamy.
- Enjoy as a refreshing and anti-inflammatory smoothie.

Nutritional value (per serving):

- Calories: 320 kcal
- Protein: 24 g
- Fat: 14 g
- Carbohydrates: 32 g
- Fiber: 8 g
- Sugar: 18 g

Cooking time: 5 minutes

Recipe 7:

Superfoods Detox Smoothie

Ingredients:

- 2 cups freshly squeezed orange juice, or equal quantity peeled and pitted oranges
- 1 unpeeled, pitted apple
- 1 ripe banana
- 3 tablespoons goji berries
- 1 teaspoon turmeric
- A pinch of pepper
- 1 teaspoon cinnamon
- 2 tablespoons tahini (you can up this to 4 tablespoons or even replace with almond butter)
- 3 brazil nuts
- 2 teaspoons fresh grated ginger

- 3 teaspoons chia seeds

Preparation:

- In a blender, combine all the ingredients and blend until smooth and frothy.
- Enjoy as a detoxifying and energizing smoothie.

Nutritional value (per serving):

- Calories: 420 kcal
- Protein: 10 g
- Fat: 18 g
- Carbohydrates: 60 g
- Fiber: 12 g
- Sugar: 36 g

Cooking time: 10 minutes

Recipe 8:

Coconut and Turmeric Latte

Ingredients:

- 1 cup of coconut milk
- 1/2 teaspoon of turmeric
- 1/4 teaspoon of cinnamon
- A pinch of black pepper
- 1 teaspoon of maple syrup

- 1/4 teaspoon of vanilla extract

Preparation:

- In a small saucepan over medium heat, whisk together the coconut milk, turmeric, cinnamon, pepper, maple syrup, and vanilla. Bring to a boil, then reduce the heat and simmer for 5 minutes, stirring occasionally.
- Enjoy as a warm and anti-inflammatory latte.

Nutritional value (per serving):

- Calories: 240 kcal
- Protein: 2 g
- Fat: 22 g
- Carbohydrates: 12 g
- Fiber: 2 g
- Sugar: 8 g

Cooking time: 10 minutes

Recipe 9:

Cacao and Maca Smoothie

Ingredients:

- 1 cup of almond milk
- 1 ripe banana

- 2 tablespoons of raw cacao powder
- 1 tablespoon of maca powder
- 1 tablespoon of almond butter
- 1 teaspoon of maple syrup
- A pinch of salt

Preparation:

- In a blender, combine all the ingredients and blend until smooth and creamy.
- Enjoy as a chocolatey and hormone-balancing smoothie.

Nutritional value (per serving):

- Calories: 360 kcal
- Protein: 10 g
- Fat: 18 g
- Carbohydrates: 46 g
- Fiber: 10 g
- Sugar: 24 g

Cooking time: 5 minutes

Recipe 10: Ginger and Lemon Tea

Ingredients:

- 4 cups of water
- 2 inches of fresh ginger, peeled and sliced
- 1/4 cup of fresh lemon juice

- 2 tablespoons of honey
- A pinch of cayenne pepper (optional)

Preparation:

- In a medium saucepan over high heat, bring the water and ginger to a boil. Reduce the heat and simmer for 15 minutes, until the ginger is infused.
- Strain the tea and stir in the lemon juice, honey, and cayenne if using.
- Enjoy as a soothing and immune-boosting tea.

Nutritional value (per serving):

- Calories: 60 kcal
- Protein: 0 g
- Fat: 0 g
- Carbohydrates: 18 g
- Fiber: 0 g
- Sugar: 16 g

Cooking time: 20 minutes

Chapter 8:

Special Occasion Recipes

1. Creamy Vegan Lasagna: Tofu ricotta, spinach, mushrooms, and a homemade tomato sauce are combined with gluten-free noodles to create this lasagna. It has a low fat content, high protein content, and no dairy. Six people may eat it after about one hour of preparation and cooking.

Ingredients:
- 9 gluten-free lasagna noodles
- 1 tablespoon of olive oil
- 1 onion, chopped
- 3 garlic cloves, minced
- 2 cups of mushrooms, sliced
- 4 cups of fresh spinach
- Salt and pepper, to taste
- 2 cups of tomato sauce
- 1/4 cup of nutritional yeast
- 2 tablespoons of fresh basil, chopped
- 1 block of firm tofu, drained and crumbled
- 2 tablespoons of lemon juice
- 1 teaspoon of dried oregano
- 1/4 teaspoon of nutmeg

- Vegan cheese, optional

Instructions:
- Preheat the oven to 180°C (350°F) and lightly grease a 9x13 inch baking dish.
- Cook the lasagna noodles according to the package directions, then drain and rinse with cold water.
- In a large skillet, heat the olive oil over medium-high heat. Add the onion and garlic and cook for about 15 minutes, stirring occasionally, until soft and golden.
- Add the mushrooms and spinach and cook for another 10 minutes, until the mushrooms are browned and the spinach is wilted. Season with salt and pepper, to taste.
- In a small bowl, stir together the tomato sauce, nutritional yeast, and basil. Set aside.
- In a food processor, blend the tofu, lemon juice, oregano, nutmeg, and a pinch of salt until smooth and creamy.
- To assemble the lasagna, spread a thin layer of the tomato sauce over the bottom of the prepared baking dish. Arrange 3 noodles over the sauce, then spread half of the tofu ricotta over the noodles. Top with half of the mushroom-spinach mixture, then another layer of sauce. Repeat with another layer of noodles, tofu ricotta, mushroom-spinach, and sauce. Finish with the remaining 3 noodles and the rest of

the sauce. Sprinkle some vegan cheese on top, if desired.

- Bake for 25 minutes, or until the cheese is melted and bubbly.

- Let the lasagna rest for 10 minutes before slicing and serving.

Nutritional value per serving (without cheese):
- Calories: 308
- Fat: 9 g
- Carbohydrates: 44 g
- Fiber: 7 g
- Protein: 18 g

2. Grain-Free Blueberry Coffee Cake: This delicious and fluffy coffee cake has luscious blueberries and a crunchy walnut topping. Rich in omega-3 fatty acids, high in fiber, and devoid of gluten, it is created using coconut flour, applesauce, and chia seeds. About 40 minutes are needed for preparation and cooking, and it serves 12 people.

Ingredients:
- 2 1/2 cups of unsweetened applesauce
- 1/2 cup of chia seeds
- 1 cup of coconut flour
- 1 teaspoon of baking soda
- 1/2 teaspoon of fine sea salt
- 1/2 cup of coconut oil, melted

- 1/4 cup of maple syrup
- 2 teaspoons of vanilla extract
- 2 cups of fresh or frozen blueberries
- 1/4 cup of chopped walnuts
- 2 tablespoons of coconut sugar
- 1/2 teaspoon of cinnamon

Instructions:

- Preheat the oven to 180°C (350°F) and line a 9x9 inch baking pan with parchment paper.
- In a large bowl, whisk together the applesauce and chia seeds. Let them sit for 10 minutes to gel.
- In a small bowl, whisk together the coconut flour, baking soda, and salt.
- Add the coconut oil, maple syrup, and vanilla to the applesauce-chia mixture and stir well.
- Gradually stir in the coconut flour mixture until well combined. Fold in 1 1/2 cups of the blueberries.
- Pour the batter into the prepared baking pan and spread it evenly. Sprinkle the remaining 1/2 cup of blueberries, the walnuts, the coconut sugar, and the cinnamon over the top.
- Bake for 25 to 30 minutes, or until a toothpick inserted in the center comes out clean.
- Let the cake cool completely in the pan before cutting into 12 squares and serving.

Nutritional value per serving:
- Calories: 254
- Fat: 16 g
- Carbohydrates: 26 g
- Fiber: 9 g
- Protein: 5 g

3. Warm Butternut Squash and Sweet Potato Salad: Quinoa, kale, roasted sweet potatoes and butternut squash, cranberries, and pumpkin seeds make up this beautiful and filling salad. You may eat it warm or cold, served with a zesty vinaigrette of lemon and mustard. Antioxidants, vitamins, and minerals abound, plus it is vegan and gluten-free. Serving four, it requires approximately sixty minutes to prepare and cook.

Ingredients:
- 1 medium butternut squash, peeled and cubed (about 4 cups)
- 1 large sweet potato, peeled and cubed (about 2 cups)
- 2 tablespoons of olive oil
- Salt and pepper, to taste
- 1 cup of quinoa, rinsed and drained
- 2 cups of vegetable broth
- 4 cups of chopped kale, ribs removed
- 1/4 cup of dried cranberries
- 1/4 cup of pumpkin seeds

- 1/4 cup of fresh parsley, chopped

For the dressing:
- 1/4 cup of olive oil
- 3 tablespoons of lemon juice
- 2 teaspoons of Dijon mustard
- 1 teaspoon of maple syrup
- 1 garlic clove, minced
- Salt and pepper, to taste

Instructions:
- Preheat the oven to 200°C (400°F) and line a baking sheet with parchment paper.
- In a large bowl, toss the butternut squash and sweet potato with the olive oil, salt, and pepper. Spread them in a single layer on the prepared baking sheet. Roast for 35 to 40 minutes, flipping halfway, until tender and golden.
- In a small pot, bring the quinoa and vegetable broth to a boil. Reduce the heat and simmer, covered, for 15 to 20 minutes, or until the quinoa is fluffy and the liquid is absorbed. Fluff with a fork and set aside.
- In a large skillet, heat some water over medium-high heat. Add the kale and cook, stirring, for about 10 minutes, until wilted and bright green. Drain and squeeze out the excess water.

- In a small bowl, whisk together all the dressing ingredients until well combined. Season with salt and pepper, to taste.
- In a large serving bowl, toss the quinoa, kale, cranberries, pumpkin seeds, and parsley with the dressing. Top with the roasted butternut squash and sweet potato. Serve warm or cold.

Nutritional value per serving:
- Calories: 589
- Fat: 29 g
- Carbohydrates: 75 g
- Fiber: 13 g
- Protein: 13 g

4. Gluten-Free Peanut Butter Cookies: These cookies have a deep peanut butter flavor with a dash of vanilla; they're chewy and soft. They are created with flax eggs, which are high in protein and fiber, vegan, and gluten-free, with oat flour and coconut sugar. They make eighteen cookies and take around twenty-five minutes to prepare and cook.

Ingredients:
- 2 tablespoons of ground flax seeds
- 6 tablespoons of water
- 1 cup of oat flour
- 1/2 teaspoon of baking soda
- 1/4 teaspoon of salt

- 3/4 cup of natural peanut butter
- 1/2 cup of coconut sugar
- 2 teaspoons of vanilla extract

Instructions:

- Preheat the oven to 180°C (350°F) and line a baking sheet with parchment paper.
- In a small bowl, whisk together the flax seeds and water. Let them sit for 10 minutes to make flax eggs.
- In a medium bowl, whisk together the oat flour, baking soda, and salt.
- In a large bowl, beat together the peanut butter, coconut sugar, and vanilla with an electric mixer until smooth and creamy.
- Add the flax eggs and mix well.
- Gradually stir in the oat flour mixture until a soft dough forms.
- Drop rounded tablespoonfuls onto the prepared baking sheet, leaving some space between them. Flatten slightly with a fork, making a crisscross pattern.
- Bake for 10 to 12 minutes, or until the edges are lightly browned.
- Let the cookies cool on the baking sheet for 5 minutes, then transfer to a wire rack to cool completely.
- Enjoy your delicious and healthy cookies!

Nutritional value per cookie:
- Calories: 131
- Fat: 7 g
- Carbohydrates: 14 g
- Fiber: 2 g
- Protein: 4 g

5. Lemon and Herb Roasted Chicken with Vegetables: This marinated chicken has a tangy lemon and herb flavor and is moist and tender. It is cooked along with potatoes, onions, and carrots to make a filling and substantial supper. It has a high iron and protein content and is devoid of dairy and gluten. It serves four people and takes around 1.5 hours to prepare and cook.

Ingredients:
- 1/4 cup of olive oil
- 1/4 cup of lemon juice
- 2 tablespoons of fresh rosemary, chopped
- 2 tablespoons of fresh thyme, chopped
- 2 teaspoons of salt
- 1 teaspoon of pepper
- 1 whole chicken (about 4 pounds), rinsed and patted dry
- 4 garlic cloves, peeled and smashed
- 1 lemon, sliced
- 4 medium carrots, peeled and cut into chunks
- 4 medium potatoes, scrubbed and cut into wedges

- 1 large onion, peeled and cut into wedges

Instructions:
- Preheat the oven to 200°C (400°F) and lightly grease a 9x13 inch baking dish.
- In a small bowl, whisk together the olive oil, lemon juice, rosemary, thyme, salt, and pepper. Set aside.
- Place the chicken in the prepared baking dish and tuck the garlic cloves and lemon slices inside the cavity. Pour half of the marinade over the chicken and rub it all over the skin. Tie the legs together with kitchen twine and tuck the wings under the body.
- In a large bowl, toss the carrots, potatoes, and onion with the remaining marinade. Arrange them around the chicken in the baking dish.
- Roast for 1 hour and 15 minutes, or until the chicken is golden and cooked through, and the vegetables are tender. Baste the chicken and vegetables with the pan juices halfway through the cooking time.
- Let the chicken rest for 10 minutes before carving and serving with the vegetables.

Nutritional value per serving:
- Calories: 654
- Fat: 34 g
- Carbohydrates: 43 g

- Fiber: 7 g
- Protein: 47 g

6. Vegan Chocolate Mousse: This mousse has a tinge of coconut flavor and a rich, creamy chocolate flavor. It is produced with vegan, gluten-free, high-antioxidant, healthy-fat ingredients such as coconut cream, cacao powder, maple syrup, and vanilla essence. It serves four people and requires about fifteen minutes to prepare and two hours to chill.

Ingredients:
- 1 can of full-fat coconut milk, refrigerated overnight
- 1/4 cup of cacao powder
- 1/4 cup of maple syrup
- 1 teaspoon of vanilla extract
- Optional toppings: fresh berries, whipped coconut cream, shaved chocolate, etc.

Instructions:
- Scoop out the solid coconut cream from the can and transfer it to a large bowl. Discard the liquid or save it for another use.
- Using an electric mixer, whip the coconut cream until fluffy and smooth, about 5 minutes.

- Add the cacao powder, maple syrup, and vanilla extract and beat until well combined and smooth, scraping down the sides of the bowl as needed.
- Divide the mousse among four small glasses or ramekins and refrigerate for at least 2 hours, or until firm.
- Enjoy your vegan chocolate mousse with any optional toppings as desired.

Nutritional value per serving (without toppings):
- Calories: 297
- Fat: 23 g
- Carbohydrates: 24 g
- Fiber: 3 g
- Protein: 3 g

7. Quinoa and Black Bean Salad with Cilantro-Lime Dressing: This salad, which includes cooked quinoa, black beans, corn, cherry tomatoes, red onion, and cilantro, is a light and cooling meal. It can be eaten as a main course or a side and is tossed with a spicy cilantro-lime vinaigrette. It has a lot of fiber, protein, and iron and is vegan and gluten-free. It cooks and prepares in around 30 minutes for 4 people.

Ingredients:
- 1 cup of quinoa, rinsed and drained
- 2 cups of water

- 1/4 teaspoon of salt
- 1 can of black beans, rinsed and drained
- 1 cup of corn kernels, fresh or frozen
- 1 cup of cherry tomatoes, halved
- 1/4 cup of red onion, finely chopped
- 1/4 cup of fresh cilantro, chopped

For the dressing:
- 1/4 cup of olive oil
- 3 tablespoons of lime juice
- 2 tablespoons of fresh cilantro, chopped
- 1 teaspoon of cumin
- 1/2 teaspoon of salt
- 1/4 teaspoon of pepper
- 1 garlic clove, minced

Instructions:
- In a small pot, bring the quinoa, water, and salt to a boil. Reduce the heat and simmer, covered, for 15 to 20 minutes, or until the quinoa is fluffy and the water is absorbed. Fluff with a fork and transfer to a large bowl. Let it cool slightly.
- Add the black beans, corn, cherry tomatoes, red onion, and cilantro to the quinoa and toss to combine.
- In a small bowl, whisk together all the dressing ingredients until well combined. Drizzle over the quinoa salad and toss to coat.

- Serve the quinoa and black bean salad at room temperature or chilled.

Nutritional value per serving:
- Calories: 433
- Fat: 20 g
- Carbohydrates: 54 g
- Fiber: 12 g
- Protein: 14 g

8. Gluten-Free Vegan Banana Bread: This bread has a crunchy walnut topping, a sweet banana flavor, and is fluffy and moist. These gluten-free, vegan, high-fiber, high-protein ingredients—oat flour, almond flour, flax eggs, and coconut sugar—go into making it. This yields one loaf and takes approximately one hour to prepare and cook.

Ingredients:
- 2 tablespoons of ground flax seeds
- 6 tablespoons of water
- 3 ripe bananas, mashed
- 1/4 cup of coconut oil, melted
- 1/4 cup of coconut sugar
- 2 teaspoons of vanilla extract
- 1 1/2 cups of oat flour
- 1/2 cup of almond flour
- 1 teaspoon of baking powder
- 1/2 teaspoon of baking soda

- 1/4 teaspoon of salt
- 1/4 cup of chopped walnuts

Instructions:
- Preheat the oven to 180°C (350°F) and lightly grease a 9x5 inch loaf pan.
- In a small bowl, whisk together the flax seeds and water. Let them sit for 10 minutes to make flax eggs.
- In a large bowl, stir together the mashed bananas, coconut oil, coconut sugar, and vanilla extract.
- In a medium bowl, whisk together the oat flour, almond flour, baking powder, baking soda, and salt.
- Add the dry ingredients to the wet ingredients and stir until well combined. Fold in the walnuts.
- Pour the batter into the prepared loaf pan and smooth the top.
- Bake for 40 to 45 minutes, or until a toothpick inserted in the center comes out clean.
- Let the bread cool in the pan for 10 minutes, then transfer to a wire rack to cool completely.
- Enjoy your gluten-free vegan banana bread.

Nutritional value per slice (assuming 10 slices per loaf):
- Calories: 256
- Fat: 14 g
- Carbohydrates: 31 g
- Fiber: 5 g

- Protein: 6 g

Conclusion

Millions of women worldwide suffer from endometriosis, a chronic illness that results in discomfort, inflammation, and infertility. Endometriosis has no known treatment, however it can be effectively managed with food changes that can enhance quality of life. Consuming anti-inflammatory, high-fiber, and nutrient-dense meals can help lessen the hormonal imbalance and inflammation that are linked to endometriosis. On the other side, you can stop the symptoms from getting worse and the growth of endometrial tissue by avoiding foods that are heavy in fat, inflammatory, and processed.

You will find many scrumptious and healthful meals in this cookbook that are appropriate for those who have endometriosis. These recipes call for healthy, readily available ingredients that may be made into vegan, dairy-free, and gluten-free dishes. You can also alter them to suit your requirements and preferences because they are flexible and adjustable. You can discover something to satiate your palate and fuel your body whether you're searching for breakfast, a snack, a main dish, or a dessert.

With any luck, this cookbook will encourage you to switch to a healthier diet that will help with your endometriosis. You may improve your health and wellbeing by changing your eating habits in a straightforward and consistent manner. Remind yourself that you deserve to live a joyful and pain-free life and that you are not alone on this journey.

Acknowledgement

Thank you for buying this book titled "Endometriosis Cookbook". We hope that you have enjoyed the recipes and learned more about how diet can help you manage your endometriosis symptoms. Your feedback is very important to us, and we would appreciate it if you could leave a positive review for this book on Amazon. By doing so, you will help other readers find this book and benefit from it as well. To leave a review, please follow these steps:

- Go to the Amazon website and sign in to your account.
- Search for "Endometriosis Cookbook" and click on the book title.

- Scroll down to the "Customer reviews" section and click on the "Write a customer review" button.
- Rate the book from 1 to 5 stars, and write a brief comment about what you liked or disliked about the book. You can also upload a photo or video of your favorite recipe if you wish.
- Click on the "Submit" button to publish your review.

Thank you for your support and kindness. We hope that this book will inspire you to adopt and adapt to a diet that is beneficial for your endometriosis. Remember that you are not alone in this journey, and that you deserve to live a happy and pain-free life. Bon appétit!